How To Fight Cancer And Win

How To Fight Cancer And Win

Scientific Guidelines and documented facts for the successful treatment and prevention of cancer and other related health problems.

William L. Fischer

Fischer Publishing Corporation
Canfield, Ohio 44406

How To Fight Cancer And Win

Scientific Guidelines and documented facts for the successful treatment and prevention of cancer and other related health problems.

ISBN: 0-915421-07-0

Library of Congress Catalog Number 86-82612

Printed in the United States of America

Dedication

I believe the preventive approach to the killing diseases is the one best hope for the future health of people everywhere. You won't find a 'miracle pill' anywhere that can magically conquer cancer overnight — not now, and probably not ever. But many important and scientifically documented strides have been taken recently in the fast-growing field of Preventive Medicine. All the preventives that have been proven in research to have sound merit are presented for your thoughtful consideration within the pages of this book. I also point an accusing finger at some of the commercial interests who are feeding the public known carcinogens by the means of some misleading advertising. What you don't know *can* hurt you.

I dedicate this book to the prevention and eradication of cancer and the other killing degenerative diseases that pervade our nation and the westernized societies of the world today.

Contents

v

Disclaimer

This book is informational only and should not be considered as a substitute for consultation with a duly-licensed medical doctor. Any attempt to diagnose and treat an illness should come under the direction of a physician. The author is not himself a medical doctor and does not purport to offer medical advice, make diagnoses, prescribe remedies for specific medical conditions or substitute for medical consultation.

While all case histories in this book are true, names have been changed or shortened to protect the identities of the persons described.

Foreword

Cancer is the second leading cause of death in the United States. In 1985 alone, cancer claimed the lives of 462,000 Americans. Of this number, 161,700 cancer deaths (35 percent) are believed to be attributable to dietary factors. Every bite of food that enters the body plays a key role in determining the degree of health we enjoy.

Dietary studies around the world have shown that excessive intake of the wrong kind of fats, particularly when coupled with an inadequate consumption of fiber, results in a higher incidence of certain cancers. Research shows that a deficiency of certain important vitamins and minerals in the diet fosters the development of cancerous tumors. It is entirely possible that simply making some sweeping changes in the national diet could dramatically reduce the number of lives lost to cancer every year.

The National Cancer Institute now recognizes the important part that the correct diet can play in an effective cancer preventive program. In their report entitled, "Diet, Nutrition, and Cancer," the NCI names healthy foods and zeros in on suspect foods. *In How to Fight Cancer And Win,* William L. Fischer details the recommendations encompassed by the NCI report with an explanation of how these foods work physiologically. He also deals with the best diet recommendations coming out of important world-wide research. This information is a real eye-opener and you'll learn some astounding facts.

William Fischer has also presented the case for bee pollen, a powerful cancer preventive, as succinctly as possible. Considering the mountain of scientific documentation that exists on the medicinal benefits of what many call "nature's perfect food," this material alone is the result of many long hours of concentrated research.

The author's main purpose in writing this book is to alert the general public to important advances in preventive medicine. A series of measures based on present medical knowledge in the fields of nutrition, oncogenes, viruses, immunology, detection, diagnosis, treatment, rehabilitation and prevention have been targeted by health authorities with the avowed aim of reducing the number of new cancer cases by

50 percent by the year 2000. In order to achieve this goal, dietary treatments should be implemented in conjunction with, when necessary, other cancer therapeutic modalities, including surgery, radiation, chemotherapy, and biological response modifier programs, all described in this book.

Although the main purpose of this book is to encourage a preventive approach to all health disorders, including cancer, you'll find a detailed review of what's going on in current research, plus both the old and new treatments favored by orthodox medicine. I personally favor preventive medicine as being the only viable approach to conquering the killer diseases forever. Once you have read through this material and understand the importance of making the necessary changes in your lifestyle, I believe you will agree.

Suffice it to say that, within these pages you will find the first comprehensive, consolidated, and concise material covering the entire scope of the cancer problem ever written especially for the layperson. It is presented in an easy-to-read and easy-to-understand manner. You won't need a dictionary at your elbow to decipher this book. All in all, this book should serve its intended audience admirably. I urge you to take this information under close consideration. It is entirely possible that your future health and happiness are at stake.

Amar Makheja, Ph.D.
Doctor of Biochemistry
The George Washington University School of Medicine
Washington, D.C.

Preface

Dear Friends,

While I was abroad doing some of the research for this book, I had the good fortune to secure some important material written by the great international oncologist, Dr. Hans Nieper. His work is well known and highly respected all over the world. In fact, I have it on good authority that Dr. Nieper's writings on cancer treatment and prevention were consulted when our own U.S. President Ronald Reagan underwent successful treatment last year for cancerous polyps discovered in his colon. Many of Dr. Nieper's revolutionary findings are reviewed in this book.

In another highlight of my month-long trip, I was favored with a great courtesy by Dr. Johanna Budwig. Dr. Budwig was kind enough to spare some of her valuable time to meet with me personally. This amazing 79 year old woman has the verve, vitality, and energy of a lady in her 50s. Although I had read much of her incredible work, I was impressed all over again by both the woman herself and the documented cures of cancer and other debilitating and killing diseases she has accomplished with a program of simple nutrition. I personally talked with some of the people she has helped when orthodox medicine could offer no successful treatment.

Dr. Budwig shared her research on linseed oil with me and I brought back the chemical and biological documentation on just how this medicinal fat works miracles within the human body, presented for your consideration in Chapter VII. Dr. Budwig is a true humanitarian in the largest sense of the word.

All in all, this was a highly successful research mission. I was very gratified at the reception I received at the hands of the many, many scientists and specialists in the various areas of expertise we examined for presentation in this book. I think we have managed to cull the best from the best minds around the world working on the cancer problem.

I was particularly struck by the informed health-consciousness of the ordinary citizen abroad. Although many times I was invited to break bread with friends, both old and new, I often took a solitary meal in the local restaurant where I was stopping in Europe. A great many of these establishments routinely place small dishes of what I first took to be the usual condiments on the table in front of the patron. I was both astounded and very pleased to find that these dishes contained raw seeds of every description! The diner could choose from among linseeds (flaxseed), poppy seeds, pumpkin seeds, chia seeds, raw almonds, and on and on. It was delightful to be able to sprinkle a selection of seeds on a salad, use some to dress a vegetable, or simply crunch and munch a handful of health while waiting to be served.

When I first ran across this little 'seed buffet' on my table, I thought it was an isolated instance and that the restaurant owner was a health buff. But, as time went on, I found that this healthful nicety was really quite commonplace. I finally struck up a conversation with the proprietor of one of the restaurants serving seeds and questioned him. He told me that it was the result of popular demand and had been established a few years back. His regular customers expected to be served a selection of seeds. He went on to say that he had tried to discontinue the practice two years ago and found that his customers complained or went elsewhere to eat.

Some informed and knowledgeable U.S. restauranteurs have adopted this idea and serve raw seeds along with the greens and vegetables in prominent display on their salad bars. As more and more Americans make known their desire to 'eat right,' this healthy practice could sweep the country!

To your very good health,
William L. Fischer

Chapter I

Cancer Explained

What It Is & What It Does

WHAT IT IS — Cancer in man is a group of related diseases (over 100) which may develop in any part of the body. Cancer can strike anyone of any age, but comes more frequently as we get older. One death in every five in the U.S. comes from cancer. Statistics show that over 66 million Americans now living will eventually develop cancer. Cancer occurs in just about three out of every four families in the United States and it kills more children between the ages of 3 and 14 than any other disease.

But a diagnosis of cancer is not necessarily a death sentence. Dr. Vincent T. DeVita, Jr., Director of the National Cancer Institute, says, "The American people are unduly pessimistic about what happens to them when they have cancer. Truly, half the cancers in this country are curable." Statistics from the N.C.I. show steady progress against this most-feared of all diseases. In the 1930s, less than 20 percent of cancer victims survived for five years. By the 1940s, the five-year rate of survival had grown to 25 percent. Today, over 50 percent of diagnosed cancer patients survive to reach the magic number of five years. Children have fared even better. At least 60 percent are expected to be among those surviving for five years.

WHAT IT DOES — How does this killer operate? In brief, *cancer is the uncontrolled and disorderly multiplication of abnormal cells which form* a malignant *tumor* (neoplasm) that

1

is usually identified medically as a *carcinoma* or *sarcoma,* depending on what part of the body is involved. The main difference between *benign* and *malignant* tumors is that benign tumors are usually enclosed within a capsule composed of a membrane of connective tissue. Benign tumors don't spread and degenerative cell changes are much less frequent than in malignant tumors.

But a cancerous cell operates outside natural law. Cancer destroys life by invading an essential organ where it grows out of control. When it expands to the point where the organ can no longer carry on its essential function, death inevitably follows. Dr. Lance Liotta, Chief of the NCI's Laboratory of Pathology, explains, "Cancer invasion and metastasis (spreading) is the main cause of treatment failure. That is really what kills the patient in most cases."

The human body is a gigantic collection of cells. Cells and the products of cells make up all the tissues and organs of the body. All bodily functions are carried on by cells. Cells of one tissue differ from those of other tissues, depending on what function they perform. The chromosomes contained in the nucleus of each cell carry the programming that determines how the cell will function in the body.

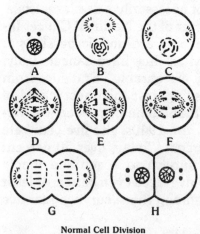

Normal Cell Division

Four phases of mitotic division in a cell having four chromosomes. A, B, C, Changes in the centrosome and nucleus during prophase. D, Metaphase. E, F, Anaphase. G, H, Telophase.

New cells develop only from preexisting cells and come into being by a process called *mitosis,* or cell division. During mitosis, the cell's chromosomes divide and move to opposite sides of the original cell. Upon completion of the last of the four phases of mitosis, each of the two new daughter cells is an exact duplicate of the original cell, complete with a full set of programmed chromosomes that tell it what to do and how to function.

ONCOGENES — This term comes from the Greek word 'onkos,' or tumor, and signifies a gene with the potential to cause a cancerous tumor. Packed into each and every cell in our body are upwards of 50,000 bits of information called genes. Genes comprise the genetic code for all parts of our bodies. Among the 50,000 genes present in each cell, science has identified about 20 different proto-oncogenes in perfectly normal genetic material. This means that every single one of us carries proto-oncogenes capable of developing into cancer.

Since proto-oncogenes are present in all normal cells, the question is *what turns them on?* Why do some unfortunate individuals develop cancer while others, even those in the same household, do not? Researchers are working overtime to target the triggers. Certain external factors (including chemicals, viruses, exposure to radiation) are being investigated because of their ability to cause gene-mutations. In connection with a Milan, Italy cancer research institute, the NCI (National Cancer Institute, Bethesda, Maryland) has conducted studies which indicate that a mutagenic agent can cause a normal cell to turn cancerous.

Since the exciting news that oncogenes have been identified, scientists all over the world are now investigating two different theories: (1) Can just one activated oncogene produce cancer?, or (2) Must multiple oncogenes be activated to produce cancer?

A cautious dissenting voice protesting the enthusiasm expressed by many scientists comes from Professor Peter H. Duesberg, Department of Molecular Biology, University of California, Berkeley. Publishing in the May 10th, 1985 issue of *Science,* Professor Duesberg says, "Despite the popularity of these hypotheses, it is pointed out here that there is as yet no convincing evidence that activated proto-oncogenes are necessary, much less sufficient, for carcinogenesis."

However, independent but related laboratory experiments undertaken by three different groups appear to confirm the theory that mutated genes do develop into cancer. Studies conducted by Robert A. Weinberg, Massachusetts Institute of Technology, and R.F. Newbold and R.W. Overell of the Institute of Cancer Research, Buckinghamshire, England, and H. Earl

3

Ruley, of the Cold Spring Harbor Laboratory in New York, support the hypothesis that at least two agents are required for a malignancy to develop. These scientists all produced cancer in their respective laboratories by treating normal genes with two carcinogenic agents.

Weinberg reported that a single cancer gene does not turn normal rat embryo cells cancerous, but that pairs of cancer genes do. Ruley's research confirmed that pairs of cancerous genes produce a malignancy, but a lone cancer gene does not. The British researchers found that newborn hamster skin cells became cancerous when treated with a carcinogenic chemical and one cancer gene, but not when treated singly with one or the other.

All in all, now that science has identified proto-oncogenes in the genetic material stored in our cells and is hot on the trail of the triggers that turn them on, certainly some optimism is justified. Once we know what turns them on, science has a good chance of developing a method of turning them off. In the meantime, avoiding known mutagenic agents just makes good sense. (See Chapter 4.)

When examined under a microscope, early cancer cells look very much like the original healthy cells from which they originated. Indeed, they may function *almost* normally for a while, with little or no symptoms to give you a clue they are planning to wreak havoc within your body. This is one reason why early detection is difficult. The body automatically repairs cellular damage in an ongoing process, but when enough harm is caused to the cell's DNA (deoxyribonucleic acid) programming, it is turned into an active oncogene and cell division goes out of control. The DNA fights damage coming from many sources, including carcinogenic (cancer-causing) chemicals in water, food, and the polluted environment, plus unavoidable cosmic radiation, ultraviolet light from the sun, radiation from diagnostic x-rays, viral infections, and random genetic alterations. On top of all that, smokers pollute both themselves and the air we all breathe with the documented carcinogens in tobacco smoke.

As the DNA begins to lose the battle and the disease progresses, the cancer cells become increasingly abnormal in appearance, structure, and function. Chromosomes in malignant cells undergoing division become oversized and many exhibit additional abnormalities showing up in a large number of different sizes and shapes. A single cell with active oncogenes divides into two abnormal cells, then four, then eight, and so on. Each cell

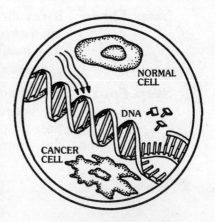

The Development of A Cancerous Cell

divides until a malignant lump (tumor) begins to form. After a period of time, which varies considerably depending on the type of cancer, the malignant cells can no longer be recognized as daughters of the original healthy cell tissue.

A comforting thought comes from Dr. Curtis Harris, Chief of the National Cancer Institute's Laboratory of Human Carcinogenesis. Dr. Harris points out that a normal cell must go through at least four distinct steps to become cancerous. As you read through these steps, outlined below, please be very much aware that we can exert considerable control over Step One.

Step One   A carcinogen (dietary factors, chemical pollutants, tobacco smoke) turns on an oncogene, the first step in preparing to make the cell cancerous.

Step Two   The cell is now medically termed *precancerous* and begins to grow more actively than a normal cell, but it is not yet a true cancer cell. (If precancerous cells are promptly identified in nonessential tissue, a physician may opt for early removal of the involved cells to prevent steps three and four from occurring.)

5

Step Three   If identification is not made and no intervening measures are instituted, another mutation may occur. When this happens, the precancerous cell evolves into true cancer.

Step Four   At this point, the cell's DNA programming has become genetically unstable and mutation progresses rapidly, resulting in the development of a malignant tumor.

If their wild multiplication is not checked, the cancer cells will freely invade and destroy neighboring tissue. A particular danger is that the malignant cells can hitch a ride and travel through the bloodstream or lymphatic system to establish a cancer colony in another part of the body. The medical term for the ability of a malignancy to spring up in another part of the body is called *metastasis*. In order to spread, cancer cells must break through the thin layer of membrane (basement lamina) which protects all tissue from invasion. Once cancer cells have broken into the bloodsteam (or have invaded a lymph node), they are carried along by the blood (or lymphatic fluid) until they become lodged in a new area. There they again tunnel through the protective membrane where they divide and multiply until a new cancer is formed.

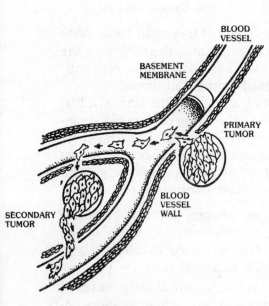

BLOOD VESSEL

BASEMENT MEMBRANE

PRIMARY TUMOR

BLOOD VESSEL WALL

SECONDARY TUMOR

Metastasis

6

How Cancer Spreads Through The Body

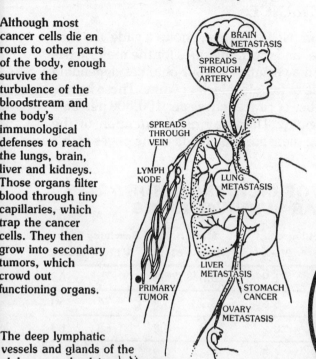

Although most cancer cells die en route to other parts of the body, enough survive the turbulence of the bloodstream and the body's immunological defenses to reach the lungs, brain, liver and kidneys. Those organs filter blood through tiny capillaries, which trap the cancer cells. They then grow into secondary tumors, which crowd out functioning organs.

BRAIN METASTASIS
SPREADS THROUGH ARTERY
SPREADS THROUGH VEIN
LYMPH NODE
LUNG METASTASIS
LIVER METASTASIS
PRIMARY TUMOR
STOMACH CANCER
OVARY METASTASIS

Routes of spread of cancer of the prostate to adjacent tissues: 1. bladder; 2. abdominal cavity; 3. rectum; 4. anal sphincters; 5. urethra. Early cancer of the prostate does not usually cause symptoms of bladder obstruction and the best hope of early discovery is rectal examination at intervals advised by a physician.

PROSTATE

The deep lymphatic vessels and glands of the abdomen and pelvis.

Kidney
Lumbar glands
Sacral glands
Internal iliac glands
Rectum
Bladder
Deep lymphatics of penis
Testicle

In some cases of malignant disease, these glands become enormously enlarged.

(Sacral glands) These and the internal iliac glands are affected in malignant disease of the *bladder, rectum* or *uterus.*

Cancer spreads throughout the body by piercing the protective membranes enclosing all tissue. It then enters the bloodstream or lymphatic system. As primary cancer cells become lodged in the tiny capillaries feeding vital organs or in the lymph passageways, they form secondary tumors. As these secondary tumors multiply and divide, they begin to encroach on the host organ. Eventually, if allowed to proliferate, the organ is so infiltrated by the tumor that it can no longer perform its essential function.

7

WHAT ARE MY CHANCES?

The table below, from NCI statistics, shows a wide variance in the five-year survival and mortality rates for the major types of cancer. There's even a variance in your chances depending on whether you're male or female, black or white. These figures are based on the number of cancer cases per 100,000 persons. Look them over carefully. Then pay close attention to the documented preventive measures you'll find in the pages of this book.

NCI SUMMARY OF INCIDENCE, MORTALITY, & 5-YEAR SURVIVAL RATES

Site/Type	Incidence		Mortality		% Surviving 5-Yrs	
	White	Black	White	Black	White	Black
Breast	85.6	71.9	26.6	26.3	75	63
Bladder	15.4	8.6	3.9	3.8	74	50
Cervix	8.8	20.2	3.2	8.8	68	63
Esophagus	2.9	11.5	2.6	9.2	5	3
Larynx	4.6	6.6	1.3	2.5	67	59
Lung	81.0	119.0	70.7	91.4	13	10
Multiple myeloma	3.4	7.9	2.4	5.0	24	27
Pancreas	8.9	13.6	8.6	11.0	3	3
Prostate	75.1	120.3	21.0	43.9	69	59
Rectum	15.0	11.7	3.5	3.5	49	37
Stomach	2.9	11.5	2.6	9.2	5	5
Uterus	25.1	13.4	2.0	2.9	88	57

WHAT CAUSES CANCER?

In the past ten years alone, science has come a long way in understanding the way cancer develops and what triggers the mutations that cause a normal cell to turn cancerous. The

National Cancer Institute says emphatically that many cancers can be prevented by making appropriate changes in our lifestyle. There are a number of areas where we have full control. By making the right choices, we can exercise a preventive effect against cancer.

ENVIRONMENT — The man-made chemical carcinogens which pollute the food chain and are present in our drinking water and air are largely unavoidable. Even the NCI notes that cleaning up the environment will require broad social actions or system changes to achieve effective controls. But you can ask your doctor if that x-ray is really necessary, and you can work with your employer to reduce your exposure to carcinogens which may be a part of your occupational hazard.

In fact, the NCI has exposure to occupational carcinogens as a preventable health hazard. Plans on the drawing board include educating both employers and employees in certain industries (asbestos, benzene, anilene dye) to the dangers and working with these companies to develop stringent safety standards. Incidentally, you should know that smokers who work in these industries are increasing their risk of developing cancer 50 times over.

GENETIC FACTORS — You have no control over the genes you were born with, but people born into a 'cancer-prone' family can still adopt healthy habits and have a good chance of escaping the disease. (See Chapter 12.)

LIFESTYLE CHOICES

The NCI points out that we have control over many factors which comprise a large part of our lifestyles. These factors include eliminating the use of tobacco, selecting preventive foods, eliminating suspect foods, reducing our exposure to sunlight, adopting healthy sex habits (and choosing a healthy partner), and practicing good personal hygiene.

SMOKING — Over 130,000 people die needlessly of cancer every year simply because they refuse to give up smoking tobacco. NCI statistics reveal that about 30 percent of all cancer deaths are directly attributable to smoking. It is a fact that those who smoke two or more packs of the 'cancer sticks' daily have a lung cancer death rate twenty-five times higher than non-smokers. In 1986, data shows that lung cancer may exceed breast cancer as the leading cause of cancer death among U.S. women for the first time. Since the early 1950s, lung cancer rates have increased 256 percent among women and 172 percent among men. In spite of the scientific evidence targeting the carcinogens in tobacco smoke as a cause of cancer, known and publicized for over twenty years, there are still close to half a million Americans (approximately one out of every three adults) who still puff away their lives — one breath at a time.

Smoking tobacco is the prime cause of both lung and laryngeal cancers, a major cause of oral and esophageal cancers, and contributes heavily to the development of bladder, kidney, and pancreatic cancers. In addition, some research indicates that a relationship between smoking and stomach, cervical, and liver cancers exists. The risk of developing cancer rises with the amount of tobacco smoked, the amount of tar exposure, and the number of years smoking has continued. Here are the frightening statistics:

Lung Cancer: In 1981 (the last year for which figures are available), 106,389 people died in the U.S. from lung cancer. Over 90 percent of lung cancer in men and 77 percent in women can be traced to cigarette smoking. When you tally up these percentages, you find that over 90,000 men and women died as a result of smoking. If you use tobacco, the odds are overwhelmingly against you.

Laryngeal Cancer: The risk of developing cancer of the larynx is 20 to 30 times higher for smokers than for nonsmokers. The major cause of laryngeal cancer is smoking. About 75 percent of the laryngeal cancer in men is attributable to tobacco smoking, compared to approximately 43 percent in women.

Oral Cancer: Projections of the mortality rate of oral cancer in tobacco users range up to thirteen times greater for smokers than for nonsmokers. This also applies to users of 'smokeless tobacco,' i.e. chewing tobacco and snuff.

Esophageal Cancer: The risk of death from esophageal cancer has been shown to be up to twelve times higher for smokers than for nonsmokers.

Other Cancers: Approximately 40 percent of the cases of *pancreatic cancer* are attributable to smoking. The risk factor for pancreatic cancer for smokers is twice that for nonsmokers. About 56 percent of the incidence of *bladder cancer* can be traced to smoking. The risk of a smoker developing *bladder cancer* is up to seven times higher than the nonsmoker. And smokers carry five times the risk of dying from *kidney cancer* as nonsmokers.

You Can't Beat the Odds: If you took your life savings to Las Vegas and played the tables against odds like these, you'd end up bankrupt. These are heavy odds to have working against you. The Surgeon General of the United States says, *"Cigarette smoking is the chief, single, avoidable cause of death in our society and the most important public health issue of our time."*

THE DIETARY FACTORS — Figures from the National Cancer Institute show that approximately 35 percent of all cancers can be attributed to dietary imbalances. Since the early 1900s, we have steadily *increased* our consumption of meat, poultry, fish, dairy products, refined sugars and sweeteners, fats and oils, and processed fruits and vegetables. We have steadily *reduced* our consumption of whole grain products, potatoes, fresh fruits and vegetables, and eggs. Let's face it. We've gotten lazy. We *like* our overprocessed chemical-saturated convenience foods.

But a vast number of studies show that excessive fat intake, inadequate dietary fiber, and a deficiency of important micronutrients (vitamins and minerals) are related to higher rates of certain cancers. (In Chapter 4, you will find an extensive review of what foods should be on the menu and what you'd be better off eliminating.) Dietary insufficiencies and excesses are associated with cancers of the gastrointestinal tract (including the esophagus, stomach, colon, rectum, pancreas, and liver), plus sex and hormone-specific sites (such as the breast, prostate, ovaries, and endometrium). Dietary factors also play a part in the development of cancers of the respiratory system and the urinary tract.

Figures Don't Lie: What we want to bring home to you here is that it's up to you to incorporate the appropriate preventive measures into your lifestyle. You don't have to smoke. And you control what you serve for dinner. The table below, prepared with hard data from the National Cancer Institute, shows very graphically that simply by eliminating tobacco and eating correctly we can reduce cancer mortality by 65 percent. And those are *good* odds to have working in your favor.

CAUSES OF CANCER DEATH

Factors Identified	Percent of Cancer Deaths
Dietary Factors	35%
Tobacco Use	30%
Sexual Behavior/Reproductive Systems	7%
Occupational Hazards	4%
Alcohol	3%
Geophysical Factors	3%
Pollution (water/food/environment)	2%
Industrial Products	1%
Medicines & Medical Procedures	1%

EARLY IDENTIFICATION VITAL

ELIMINATING THE HANDICAP — Early identification is the single greatest problem in the medical treatment of a malignancy. If cancers stayed where they began and didn't grow and spread, most malignant tumors could be successfully treated. For instance, in the case of a localized cancer, the five-year survival rate is well over 80 percent. However, if the exact same type of tumor invades the lymph nodes, which have pathways all over the body, the five-year survival rate drops to around 32 percent. Only 1.2 percent of persons with metastasized (spreading) cancers survive for five years.

Quite obviously, the medical treatment of an early *prime* (original) cancer is many times more successful, and less drastic, than the treatment required for cancer which has spread (metastasized) from its original site to other parts of the body. Many scientists believe more than half of all cancers can be completely cured if identified in their early stages. Early detection and prompt effective treatment is essential.

DIAGNOSTIC TECHNIQUES

EARLY DETECTION — There are a number of common medical techniques which allow doctors to detect and diagnose an early malignancy. Even more non-invasive diagnostic aids are being developed by scientists around the world. Very soon, a biopsy, in which the surgeon takes a cutting of suspect tissue for microscopic examination, may be a thing of the past. Here's a quick review of the most common methods of detection.

Cervical Cancer: One of the easiest and most effective techniques for detecting cervical cancer in women is the Pap test. By examining the cells naturally sloughed off by the uterus, the physician can identify a potentially dangerous precancerous condition, or an existing malignancy, and initiate prompt treatment. Data shows that death from cervical cancer is on the decline, but is still far from a rare occurrence, especially among black women.

Bladder Cancer: Cells that are shed by the bladder into the urine may indicate the presence of early bladder cancer. Certain groups at high risk of developing bladder cancer, such as workers in the aniline-dye industry, are routinely screened by this method.

Breast Cancer: Mammography, a special x-ray technique, can detect breast cancers as tiny as two-tenths (0.2) of an inch, much too small to be felt. Another new procedure, *thermography,* records the heat patterns of the breast and allows the physician to note the pattern characteristic of early cancer. It is important to note here that statistics show that regular breast examinations, including screening with mammography, have led to a reduction in deaths due to breast cancer, not only over the short term, but in the long run as well. A survey conducted by the NCI revealed that only one out of every five women surveyed reported ever having had a mammogram.

The NCI is out to change these statistics. The experts say that annual screening would result in a 30 percent reduction in breast cancer mortality.

One final note: After all the controversy over the relationship of oral contraceptives to breast cancer, data coming from an extensive Swedish study and Norwegian study (as published in the prestigious British publication, *Lancet*, September 1986) appears to be conclusive. We quote from pertinent passages: "We found no statistically significant association between the use of oral contraceptives for 7 completed years or less with premenopausal breast cancer. However, our data for the long-term use of oral contraceptives beyond 7 years and particularly for 12 years or more are suggestive of an association with an increased risk of premenopausal breast cancer. The duration of oral contraceptive use before the first full-term pregnancy and the total duration of use correlated strongly in our series." In other words, young women who use oral contraceptives before their first-term pregnancy are just as much at risk of developing breast cancer as are women who take the pill for 12 years or more. If you refuse to give up this popular form of birth control (and many of you will prefer to take your chances), it is doubly important that you regularly monitor your breasts for lumps and have regular screenings by your physician.

Colorectal Cancer: Unfortunately, the early detection of colorectal cancer by means of a proctoscopic examination has not been popular among the general public and few physicians employ this means of examination on a routine basis. If you value your life and health, you might want to consider having an annual proctoscopic exam after the age of forty.

Sam Shapiro, B.S., past director of the Health Services Research & Development Center (Baltimore, Maryland) and Professor Emeritus, School of Public Health, Johns Hopkins University (Baltimore, Maryland) points out that "There is a strong conviction in many circles that a public education program, accompanied by elevated professional attention, is needed to increase knowledge about risk factors and receptivity to messages about diet, improve responsiveness to symptoms, and increase the frequency of proctoscopy performance as part of general physical examinations starting for those in the middle years of life."

Lung Cancer: A technique similar to the Pap test can be used to verify a suspected lung cancer long before it is large enough to appear on an x-ray. A microscopic examination of cells taken from the surface of the oral cavity can assist in identifying early mouth and throat cancer.

Oral Cancer: You might not even be aware that your dentist looks for the tell-tale early warning signs of oral cancer while he's poking around your mouth with his instruments. Oral cancer cases are on the increase. In 1985, close to 30,000 new cases were discovered in the U.S., more than double the cases reported in 1970. Science says that tobacco (especially cigarettes and chewing tobacco), alcohol, syphilis, and bad oral hygiene are the major contributing factors. In addition, new studies indicate that the herpes simplex virus and a chronic iron deficiency increase oral cancer risk.

Your dentist is an able diagnostician of oral cancer. But the problem is that we don't always see our dentist often enough. The elderly, at high risk of developing oral cancer, go to their medical doctor six times more often than they go to the dentist. Statistics show that half of those age 65 or older have not seen a dentist in five or more years. For those age 65 or older who wear dentures, more than seventy percent have not seen a dentist in five years or more.

In every 100,000 persons, 7.5 will die from oral cancer. Probably because more men than women chew tobacco and drink, the breakdown is 5.6 men in every 100,000, compared to 1.9 women. Three-quarters of these deaths are in persons 55 years of age and older. The five-year survival rate is low (30-35%), possibly because half of the oral cancers have metastasized before being discovered.

Drs. G.T. Chiodo, T. Eigner, and D.I. Rosenstein, publishing in *Postgraduate Medicine* (August 1986) believe that once primary care physicians routinely screen for oral cancer, survival rates will improve. They say, "Prognosis improves vastly when the lesion is detected and treated early. One study has demonstrated a 64 percent five-year survival rate for patients with oral cancer that was diagnosed before regional lymph node involvement versus a 15 percent five-year survival rate for patients whose lesions were diagnosed after metastasis. By including an oral cancer examination in routine physical examination of patients, the physician and public health nurse can increase the likelihood of early detection of oral cancer." In the meantime, the bottom line is that you should see your dentist twice a year, and not just to have your teeth cleaned either.

LOOKING AHEAD

The National Cancer Institute has developed a comprehensive program aimed at substantially reducing the number of cancer cases in the nation by the year 2000. A detailed plan entitled *Cancer Control — Objectives for the Nation — 1985 to 2000* has already been implemented. The following table summarizes these objectives and what the NCI is doing about them. The following statement comes from this landmark NCI report: *"On the basis of current knowledge alone, the NCI estimates that, at a minimum, 30,000 lives could be saved in the year 2000 if Americans would modify their dietary habits."* The key to the success (or failure) of this grand goal is you and me and every citizen of the U.S. We have the knowledge to make it work. All we have to do is follow the plan and incorporate these recommendations in our lives.

MEDICAL PROCEDURES

TYPE OF CANCER DETERMINES TREATMENT — The successful medical treatment of cancer requires the complete removal or destruction of all malignant tissue. The first line of defense is surgery. For surgery to provide a cure for cancer, the operation must be performed before the malignancy has spread into organs and tissues that sustain life.

The choice of medical treatment against cancer is governed by the type, location, and size of the tumor at the time of diagnosis. Surgery, radiation, chemotherapy, drug and hormone treatments, laser and heat therapies, interferon, anti-

THE NCI CANCER CONTROL OBJECTIVES

Action	Target	Rationale	Year 2000 Objectives	Estimated Death Reduction
Prevention	Smoking	The relationship between smoking and cancer has been scientifically established.	Reduce percentage of adults who smoke from 34% (in 1983) to 15% or less. Reduce percentage of youths who smoke by age 20 from 36% (in 1983) to 15% or less.	8 to 15%
	Diet	Research shows that high-fat low-fiber consumption may increase risk for various cancers. Studies have persuaded the NCI to recommend an increase in fiber. New research is underway to verify the relationships and test the impact on cancer incidence.	Reduce average consumption of fat from 38% to 30% or less of total calories. Increase average consumption of fiber from 8-12 grams to 20-30 grams daily.	8%
Screening	Breast	The effectiveness of breast screening in reducing mortality has been scientifically established.	Increase percentage of women aged 50-70 who have an annual breast exam coupled with mammography from 45% to 80% for physical exam and 15% for mammography.	3%
	Cervix	The effectiveness of cervical screening in reducing mortality has been scientifically established.	Increase percentage of women who have a Pap smear every 3 years from 79% (ages 20-39) to 90% and from 57% (ages 40-70) to 80%.	3%
Treatment	Put research results into practice.	NCI review of certain trials and data shows that (for certain cancer sites) mortality is greater than experienced in clinical trials.	Increase adoption of state-of-the-art treatment.	10 to 14%
Treatment		With accelerated gains in state-of-the-art treatment.		26%
Total Range of Mortality (Death-Rate) Reduction by Year 2000				25 to 50%

bodies, and the special knowledge of oncogenes, are some of the cancer-fighting methods available to the treating physician.

Often the busy physician is unable to take the time needed to really sit down with a patient and explain what the projected therapy is designed to do and what to expect. But a thorough understanding of the procedure goes a long way toward reassuring the patient and helps make the treatment a thousand times more bearable.

In this book, under the heading of *Scientific Discoveries,* we examine the various medical treatments currently in use against cancer, or just over the horizon. In non-technical language, we explain exactly how the newest methods work, how well they work (or don't work), and how they affect the body. We report on the latest developments in cancer research and let you in on the progress the scientists are making.

In the segment entitled *Nutritional & Holistic Treatments,* you are introduced to certain common nutrients that many authorities believe can strengthen the body against cancer. We examine the macrobiotic diet and explain why it may be a possible cancer-preventive. Another effective technique explored under this heading is visualization therapy. This method has worked for many against varied conditions of ill health, including cancer. Finally, we report on a vitally important dietary supplement from Europe which scientists deservedly call a real breakthrough in the fight against cancer and other life-threatening conditions.

BE INFORMED

A WIDE VARIETY OF INFORMATION — This book is a serious effort to bring you information which may ease your mind by explaining the treatment your doctor judges best for medically treating an existing malignancy. Perhaps even more important is the material on the possible cancer-fighting nutritional and holistic methods you can put into practice yourself.

In this polluted world we live in, staying healthy is almost a full-time job. The knowledgeable, self-educated individual who takes the time to stay informed on the important advances in health care and preventive medicine has a better chance than most of enjoying good health into his sunset years.

The World of Science & Medicine
A Brief Review

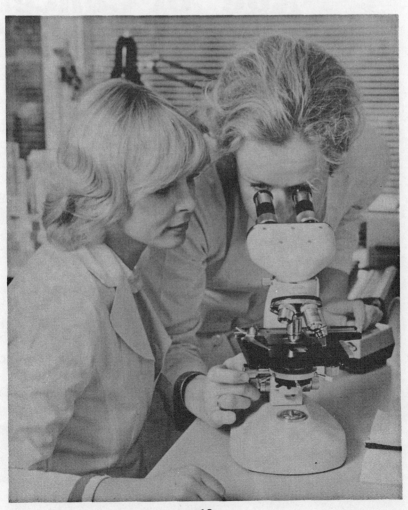

Chapter II

Is this the "Golden Age" of Cancer Research?

In the Footsteps of a Killer

Science is beginning to take some giant strides in the quest for knowledge about what causes cancer and how best to treat it. Once science is able to pinpoint exactly how cancer develops within the body and what makes a perfectly normal cell go haywire and turn malignant, the medical community has a good chance of discovering how to beat it. Until that long-awaited day arrives, prevention remains the key and that is the basic thrust of this book.

STATISTICALLY SPEAKING

If we look only at the numbers, it certainly looks like science is winning the war against cancer. For instance, it is a fact that people diagnosed as having malignant tumors are living longer than they did ten years ago. But one of the problems involved in accepting some of the optimistic cancer survival statistics as gospel is termed the *staging effect*.

Here's how it works: Using all the diagnostic resources at his command, when an oncologist brings in a definite diagnosis of a malignancy, he is able to define what *stage* the cancer is in. Under the staging system, a cancer is labeled either Stage I (early), Stage II (growing) or Stage III (advanced).

More and more Stage I tumors are being discovered today because more and more people are paying attention to their health, and also because diagnostic procedures have become more precise. Now that science can more easily detect metastases (spreading), a tumor which would have been categorized as Stage I some years ago is now tagged Stage II. Let's say that these statistics are fed into a waiting computer and correlated with data from all over the country.

What happens is this: As a group, Stage I patients will *appear* to have gained an increased life expectancy, but only because their tumors were discovered many months earlier and precise diagnosis led to the exclusion of patients in Stage II who would have been labeled Stage I ten years ago. The survival rate of Stage I patients is technically improved by very early diagnosis and by the absence of Stage II patients. The survival rate of the Stage II group is also automatically improved because a decade ago their metastases would not have been detected. So, looking only at the data, both groups appear to live longer, not, unfortunately, because of advancements in treatment, but because of the staging effect phenomenon caused by earlier and more precise diagnosis.

Let's look at a mythical patient with an inoperable and medically untreatable cancer who would have been given only six months to live after being diagnosed ten years ago. Today, due to better diagnostic procedures, let's say his cancer is detected 12 months earlier than would have been possible a decade ago. *Statistically speaking, he now has an increased life expectancy because he has 18 months to live.* His increased life expectancy is not because medical science is now able to alter the course of his disease, but because it was diagnosed a year earlier. In actuality, this patient is no better off right now than he was ten years back.

In his landmark paper entitled, "Progress Against Cancer?" published in the *New England Journal of Medicine* (May 1986), John C. Bailar, Ph.D. (Harvard School of Public Health, Boston, Massachusetts) makes some disturbing points.

Dr. Bailar is calling for an open debate to evaluate the progress science is making against this dread disease and to determine how best to proceed. Dr. Bailar notes, "In 1962, cancer was the recorded cause of death for 278,562 Americans. In 1982, just 20 years later, 433,795 persons died of cancer—a 56 percent increase . . . From 1973 to 1981, the crude incidence rate for all cancers combined rose by 13 percent and the age-adjusted incidence rate by 8.5 percent."

Dr. Bailar says emphatically, "The sharp and continuing rise in deaths from lung cancer, nearly all from cigarette smoking, is now widely recognized as a medical, social, and political scandal." (The April 1986 issue of the *Congressional Quarterly* says that over 500 million tax dollars will be spent over the next five years to prop up tobacco prices.) See the following chart.

CANCER DEATHS PER 100,000
1950 Through 1982
In The Total U.S. Population

Dr. Bailar continues, (As the chart shows), "Mortality from cancer of the prostate has not changed appreciably in the entire male population. Mortality from stomach cancer has steadily declined, relecting changes in incidence rather than better methods of treatment, earlier diagnosis, or changes in definition. Mortality from cervical cancer has declined dramatically as a result of wide-spread screening programs, improved standards of living, and a high rate of hysterectomy. The incidence of breast cancer shows a peak in 1974 and a slower rise in more recent years. Finally, mortality from cervical cancer has also declined slowly and steadily."

The following table shows very graphically that the five-year survival rates for various cancers have not changed appreciably in the years from 1973 through 1978, the last year for which data is available.

PERCENT OF CANCER VICTIMS SURVIVING FOR FIVE YEARS AFTER DIAGNOSIS

Year:	1973	1974	1975	1976	1977	1978
All Cancers	38.5	40.6	41.0	41.2	40.8	40.1
Colorectal Cancer	36.2	37.8	38.2	39.6	39.4	38.7
Lung Cancer	9.0	9.8	9.7	10.3	10.6	11.0
Breast Cancer	64.3	65.2	67.0	66.0	66.0	65.0
Prostate Cancer	41.2	43.9	45.9	47.7	47.8	47.4
Hodgkin's Disease	57.7	63.3	66.6	71.9	69.5	67.3

Dr. Bailar says, "We see no reason for optimism about overall progress during recent years. There is no reason to think that, on the whole, cancer is becoming any less common. Data provides no evidence that some 35 years of intense and growing efforts to improve the treatment of cancer have had much overall effect on the most fundamental measure of clinical outcome — death. With respect to cancer as a whole, we have slowly lost ground. Overall, the effort to control cancer has failed — so far — to attain its objectives."

To understand Dr. Bailar's statements, which certainly reflect his concern over our failure to conquer the cancer problem, please see the following chart. And, before you despair, be aware that documented preventive measures against cancer exist and are clearly spelled out in later chapters in this book.

CASES OF ALL TYPES OF CANCER FROM 1973 THROUGH 1981
Rates Shown Are Per 100,000 Population
U.S. Population

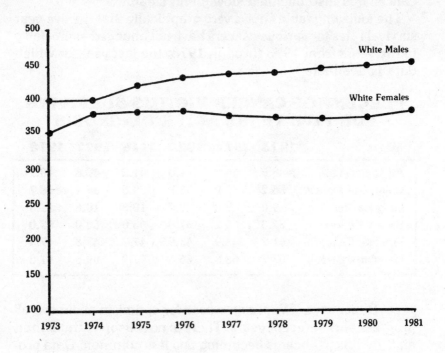

Critics say that the mortality rates from cancer are not truly indicative of the overall picture because they include the continually escalating rise of death from lung cancer. Taking this argument into consideration, Dr. Bailar found that the death rate from 1950 to the present shifts down from an 8 percent increase when lung cancer rates are figured in to a satisfying 13 percent decrease when lung cancer rates are left out. Carrying his calculations even further, Dr. Bailer excluded the rates for cancer of the stomach and cervix because, as he points out, these rates have also been changing, but not because of any advancement in the method of treatment. What he found clinched his argument. Dr. Bailar notes, "The age-adjusted mortality then shifts from 130.1 in 1950 to 128.9 in 1980 — a change of less than one percent. It is difficult to claim success in the war against cancer based on these figures."

What this means to you and me is that our chances of surviving cancer today are really no better than they were thirty years ago — unless we take matters into our own hands and incorporate the documented preventive measures into our lifestyle.

However, in the meantime, scientists all over the world are working overtime to develop and perfect the treatments that may lead to our ability to cure cancer. Medical science says that a lot of promising developments in the treatment of cancer are just over the horizon. Here's what's going on.

CLUES TO TREATMENTS OF THE FUTURE

In this chapter, we're going to bring you up-to-date on the undeniably solid developments coming out of current scientific research. Frank Rauscher, Jr., Senior Vice President of the American Cancer Society, has been quoted as saying, "We are now in the golden age of cancer research. Although we most likely won't cure or prevent most cancers by the end of the decade, there's a good chance we can do it by the end of the century." Here's what's going on.

BIOLOGICAL MODIFIERS
Some new compounds attempt to convert cancer cells into normal ones. Others try to stimulate the body's immune system. And monoclonal antibodies, custom-made proteins similar to the body's natural defenders, may one day carry poisons directly to tumor cells.

BIOLOGICAL RESPONSE MODIFIERS — According to the National Cancer Institute, biological response modifiers appear very promising. The basic premise here is to stimulate (or restore) the body's own defenses so that all the potentially lethal anticancer forces of the body are mobilized and strengthened for the internal fight. All over the world, scientists are investigating ways to program the immune system to resist cancer and other diseases as well.

In the early 1980s, the NCI established BRMP (The Biological Response Modifiers Program) to identify and study new biological materials which fight cancer. Since that time,the BRMP researchers have identified hundreds of chemical substances which can influence the normal defenses of the body. Several groups of biological materials which are believed to be clinically important are currently being studied and tested.

THE IMMUNE SYSTEM — It is by producing antibodies and immune cells that the internal police system of the body fights disease. Antibodies, proteins which actively attack abnormal cells, and special white blood cells work within the immune system to surround and devour both diseased cells and viral invaders. *Macrophages* are the scavengers that gobble up foreign cells. The good news is that it has been determined that some chemical agents may be able to activate the macrophages, thereby stimulating the immune defense against malignant cells. Research is continuing.

INTERLEUKIN-2 — Steven Rosenberg, M.D. Ph.D., the Chief of Surgery at the NCI in Bethesda, Maryland has

26

achieved what he himself cautiously calls a major breakthrough in man's continuing fight against cancer. Dr. Rosenberg says, "It's not a cancer cure in 1985, but it is a breakthrough in that it marks the first successful approach to using the body's own immune system to reject a cancer."

Interleukin-2 is a complex protein genetically programmed to boost the body's own white blood cells' ability to fight cancer. This space-age immunotherapy treatment involves hooking up the patient to cell-separating equipment which identifies and isolates a portion of the body's white blood cells. These disease-fighting cells, already a part of the vital immune system, are then mixed with interleukin-2 before they are returned to the bloodstream for their search and destroy mission.

The success of interleukin-2 is far from 100 percent. In the group of 25 patients accepted in the initial study, Dr. Rosenberg's NCI team reports that 11 patients had a 50 percent shrinkage in the size of their malignant tumors, but 14 patients did not respond and are still listed as terminal.

Although immunotherapy patients develop severe side effects, these effects are reversed at the close of the month-long treatment. Side effects include a weight-gain of up to 30 pounds because of fluid retention, which may lead to lung, kidney and liver disorders, plus flu-like symptoms such as chills, fever and diarrhea. Because patients accepted in the NCI program (only eight can be treated each month) are individuals who have not responded to conventional treatment and who are considered terminal, the side effects of interleukin-2 are risks most are eager to take.

Even though less than half of the patients involved in the clinical trials with interleukin-2 have responded favorably so far, medical science believes that further refinements of this immunotherapy program will increase the success rate considerably. Trials are continuing.

INTERFERON — Cancer research centers all over the globe, including six in the U.S., are studying interferon in clinical trials on human patients. The aim is to discover the maximum safe dosage, the quantity where maximum effect occurs, the best schedule of administration, and any possible toxic effects. In correlating the data, the NCI reports limited success and states that interferon is clearly beneficial in some respects.

A 50 percent reduction in tumor size has been documented in some few patients with breast cancer, melanoma, and other solid tumors. Results achieved in patients with kidney cancer were more promising and more than half of the leukemia patients involved responded favorably to interferon therapy. Side effects observed in patients include chills, fever, fatigue, decreased white blood cell count and abnormal liver function. However, when the interferon therapy was withdrawn, the side effects usually disappeared.

The theory here is that although interferon is not lethal to cancer, it apparently can slow malignant growth so that the cancerous cells no longer multiply and will eventually die. Laboratory studies with animals indicate that a combination of interferon and an anticancer drug may be more effective than using interferon alone. Research is proceeding on the theory that interferon will probably prove to be most useful in connection with other types of conventional cancer treatment.

AMPLIGEN — Ampligen, developed by scientists at John Hopkins University in Baltimore, is a highly promising biological response modifier. Because of its chemical formula, Ampligen is subject to enzymatic action in the blood and decomposes rapidly, but not before accomplishing its purpose. Because of this feature, Ampligen is less toxic than some of the other compounds under study as biological response modifiers. Ampligen also differs from some of the other drugs under investigation in that it doesn't stimulate the body's immune system to produce antibodies against it.

TUMOR NECROSIS FACTOR — TNF, or the tumor necrosis (killing) factor, is a substance (protein) produced naturally by *macrophages,* the white blood cells of the immune system that gobble up dangerous invaders. Tests in laboratory animals show that TNF acts directly on the defenses of the body by stimulating protective lymphocytes and macrophages. Researchers in both the U.S. and Japan have artificially produced TNF and trials in humans are scheduled, but the scientists agree it will be several years before TNF is approved for widespread use.

LIPOPHILIC MOLECULES — Lipophilic molecules bind with lipids (fats) in membranes. Researchers at the Dana-Farber Cancer Institute, affiliated with the prestigious Harvard Medical School (Cambridge, Massachusetts) have discovered that these charged compounds are released from normal cells, but remain active in carcinomas. Because carcinomas comprise 85 percent of human cancers, this is a very important finding.

Once a lipophilic molecule takes up residence in a cancer cell, it destroys the cell's ability to absorb enzymes necessary to its biochemical processes. These compounds have effectively inhibited the growth of human colon-carcinoma cells surgically implanted in laboratory mice. The lipophilic molecules currently being tested include *dequalinium* (an antibacterial agent), *rhodamine-123* (a dye used to change the color of laser light), and another compound used in industrial inks which has shown itself ten times more potent than dequalinium. The side effects observed in animals so far have been negligible.

HYDRAZINE — One of the truly awful effects of an advanced cancer is *cachexia*, a process of gradual starvation. Because a malignancy interferes with the normal metabolic process, the result is that the tumor absorbs the nutrients and the food consumed does not benefit the patient. Recent research indicates that in patients given hydrazine, an inexpensive and common industrial chemical, weight loss has been halted, even though their cancers were well advanced. The American Cancer Society has ordered a two-year study, now commencing its second year, on the action of hydrazine in patients with colorectal cancers.

LIGHT TREATMENT — Speaking at the American Cancer Society seminar in mid-1985, Dr. Richard Edelson of Columbia University described his process for treating blood outside the body with a drug (psoralen) which is activated by ultraviolet light. Edelson's light treatment, called *extracorporeal photophoresis* (extra [outside] corporeal [physical body] photo [Greek 'light'] phoresis [the migration of charged ions through a membrane]), involves injecting the patient with psoralen which is known to attack defective immune cells. Because psoralen is activated only by untraviolet light, two hours after administration of the drug, a portion of the patient's blood supply is removed and the white blood cells are isolated. The psoralen-saturated white blood cells are then exposed to ultraviolet radiation for less than a second and the activated blood is returned to the patient.

The Columbia University group has treated 11 patients suffering from a particularly deadly form of cancer (cutaneous T cell lymphoma) which allows its victims an average survival time of only three to five years. Two of the 11 patients have been able to discontinue treatment and remain free of cancer. Eight have shown a marked decrease in the lethal T cells.

Edelson cautions that extracorporeal photophoresis is not a cure, explaining that it eliminates some of the T cells, but doesn't stop the body from producing them altogether. Edelson says, "What we are really after is the treatment of immune diseases. I think the future for immunotherapy is very bright. In combination with other therapies, this approach may lead to good control of cancer."

In autoimmune diseases, the immune system itself goes off track and attacks the body. It is speculated that Edelson's combination drug and light therapy may also prove useful in the treatment of rheumatoid arthritis and lupus.

LASERS — In a process called *photodynamic therapy,* scientists are using an innovative combination of drugs and the laser beam to destroy cancerous growths. A non-toxic drug is administered which sensitizes cancerous lesions to light. After three days, a laser beam is directed on the tumor for 8 to 10 minutes.

The Roswell Park Memorial Institute (Buffalo, New York) has reported preliminary testing of over 3,000 cancer patients suffering with lung or bladder cancer treated by this new therapy has given some encouraging results. Between 25 to 35 percent of the patients in this study were tumor-free thirty days after treatment.

HYPERTHERMIA — A modified food-warming oven consisting of a chamber that produces radiant heat up to 108 degrees Fahrenheit appears to enhance the benefits of chemotherapy and radiation without adding further toxic side effects.

Trials conducted at the University of Wisconsin Medical School by H. Ian Robins used heat therapy on cancer patients suffering from a number of different forms of cancer. In this procedure, Dr. Robins brought the body temperature of his patients up to 107.4 degrees F. and maintained temperature for up to three hours. He reports four patients with lymphoma had a favorable response to a combination of radiation therapy and the hyperthermia technique.

Dr. Robins explains, "The advantage of whole-body hyperthermia is that it gets at disseminated cancer and boosts the beneficial effects of both chemotherapy and radiation."

CANCER-SPECIFIC AGENTS

MONOCLONAL ANTIBODIES — Monoclonal antibodies (MABs) are artificial antibodies laboratory produced to search out and destroy specific cancers. An important feature of MABs is that their destructive effect can be increased by impregnating them with a powerful anticancer drug before injecting them into the body. Because the lethal anticancer drugs currently used in chemotherapy are not cancer-specific but also destroy normal cells, this particular line of scientific endeavor may prove to be the most exciting yet.

The Scripps Clinic & Research Foundation in La Jolla, California has used MABs successfully against human tumors which were established by transplantation into lab mice. A patient in his mid-60s suffering from lymph cancer was treated at Stanford University with MABs. The treatment completely destroyed the malignancy. Children with leukemia given MAB therapy at the Dana Farber Cancer Institute have also benefited.

The most comprehensive study of MAB therapy comes from Dr. Hilary Koprowski, Director of the Wistar Institute of Anatomy & Biology in Philadelphia. Dr. Koprowski has

31

revealed results of a study of 50 cancer victims given monoclonal antibodies after they had failed to benefit from conventional treatment. Follow-ups from two to four years after the MAB therapy showed that two patients were free of any malignancy; in ten patients, the normal progress of the disease was permanently slowed; and in 25 other victims, there was at least a temporary beneficial response.

MABs may also prove to be an extremely valuable diagnostic tool. A cancer-specific MAB impregnated with a radioactive substance and then given intravenously will travel to minute cancer cells wherever they are located within the body. By scanning with special equipment, cancer can be detected by this method before conventional diagnostic methods are able to distinguish any tiny malignancy.

IMMUNOTOXINS — The production of a safe cancer-specific immunotoxin is accomplished by injecting cancer cells into a laboratory mouse. The mouse's immune system then produces antibodies having the ability to bind with the antigen site on the cancer cells. A toxin (which may be bacterial, botanical, or chemical) is added. This produces an immuno-toxin antibody with the ability to bind to the antigen on the cancer cell and destroy it. The cancer-specific immunotoxin cannot bind with the antigen site of normal cells and they are bypassed.

Although the concept appears simple and laboratory tests are promising, a number of questions must be answered before doctors are willing to risk injecting an immunotoxin directly into the body. The immunotoxin must be safe for normal tissue, stable within the body's very complex environment, and cancer-specific.

To avoid any potentially unknown destructive complications, Dr. Daniel Vallera, University of Minnesota Medical School, is studying the effect of treating bone marrow cells outside the body with immunotoxins. Conventional treatment of patients with bone cancer and leukemia often includes chemotherapy and whole-body radiation treatment, which destroys normal cells in the bone marrow which are the vital precursors of all blood cells. By using immunotoxins outside the body, Vallera demonstrated their effectiveness with minimum destruction of normal cells. The benefits of treating bone marrow in this way are now being cautiously tested on patients.

Experiments injecting immunotoxins directly into the bloodstream of a guinea pig with liver cancer conducted by Michael Bernhard of the NCI and his associates met with limited success. The group reported that a single injection shrank the tumor, but did not completely destroy it.

The hope is that a number of immunotoxins can be developed with each specific against the different types of cancer cells, but safe for normal cells. Many researchers are working on doing just that.

CANCER VACCINES — Results from an on-going study begun in 1981 by Michael G. Hanna and H. C. Hoover under the auspices of Litton Bionetics, Inc., Rockville, Maryland, indicate that a cancer vaccine might soon be a reality. Twenty cancer patients were given injections of their own malignant cells after colorectal tumor surgery. The cancer cells were first treated with radiation so that they could not reproduce and a total of three vaccinations, the first two combined with an immune system enhancer, were given each patient.

All twenty of the vaccinated patients experienced good results. None has died and only four suffered a recurrence of cancer. On the other hand, twenty colorectal cancer patients operated on at approximately the same time, but not given the vaccine, did not fare so well. Four have died of cancer and another five have recurring malignancies.

At the Roswell Park Memorial Institute in Buffalo, Heinz Kohler is working to develop an anti-idiotype vaccine which he believes will destroy the body's tolerance to a tumor. Kohler explains, "The immune system identifies shapes, but doesn't care what's behind those shapes. The idiotype provides an antibody that could be a substitute for the original antigen."

Dr. Kohler estimates that human studies are at least two or three years away, but hopes to have a vaccine ready to begin animal trials by the middle of 1986.

CONTROLLING METASTASIS — Finding a way to keep a

cancer localized and prevent *metastasis* (spreading) to another area of the body is a dream of oncologists all over the world. Researchers at the Georgetown University School of Medicine (Washington, D.C.) believe they have taken an important first step in doing just that. They appear to have discovered the way in which malignant cells escape a localized tumor and travel to another site.

A protein called *fibronectin* is a part of what holds both normal cells and cancerous cells together. When the connecting fibronectin breaks down in a cancerous cell, the malignant cell is freed and enters the bloodstream or lymphatic system where it can migrate throughout the body. Using chicken embryo cells infected with RSV (Rous sarcoma virus), which causes a cancer of the connective tissue in chickens, the scientists determined that a viral enzyme (*pp60src,* a product of RSV's cancer-causing gene), degraded the fibronectin holding the cancer cells together and allowed them to float free. The researchers concluded that without the viral enzyme, the fibronectin would remain intact. With its fibronectin intact, a cancer cell would be held in place and could not metastasize elsewhere in the body.

AS THINGS STAND NOW

It's all very good and well to look forward to a future when a 'magic bullet' containing a cancer-specific agent may possibly be developed which will kill and destroy a malignancy without harming normal tissue. In the meantime, the medical community must fight cancer with the limited means at their command. The following chapter describes the medical approach to the treatment of cancer as things stand now.

Chapter III
Orthodox Medical Treatment
Surgery, Radiation, & Chemotherapy

As science works overtime attempting to discover less damaging treatments, procedures, and chemical drugs which are cancer-specific and not toxic to normal cell tissue, medical oncologists and surgeons are fighting back with the only weapons in their arsenal.

According to the U.S. Department of Health & Human Services, 20 percent of those diagnosed as having cancer are in a stage too far advanced to be termed 'curable.' In the remaining 80 percent (those who stand a chance of a complete cure or permanent remission of the disease), surgery is the treatment of choice in 45 percent. In an additional 10 percent, surgery combined with radiation therapy is the primary method of attack.

Radiation alone is given in approximately 20 percent of the cases diagnosed. Less than 10 percent of those suffering from cancer receive chemotherapy as their first form of treatment. However, chemotherapy is considered useful for the large number of cancer victims who suffer a recurrence of some form of this dread disease.

EARLY WARNING SYSTEM

The entire health-care industry is now engaged in some important changes in the way both primary (preventive) measures and secondary (screening) controls against cancer are being handled. A massive preventive campaign has been launched by the National Cancer Institute in order to reduce the incidence of cancer cases by the year 2000. (See Chapter 14.) There's been a spurt of growth in the number of health maintenance organizations (HMOs) recently and many hospitals have expanded their outpatient facilities as well. It's easier now than it's ever been to catch cancer in its early stages. The experts say that early detection is the key to a complete cure.

In an address before the American Society of Preventive Oncology (April, 1985), Sam Shapiro, B.S., of the Health Services Research & Development Center (Baltimore, Maryland) showed the importance of detecting a malignancy in its earliest form by explaining the progress against three different cancers (breast, cervix, colorectal).

Breast Cancer — Under the auspices of the National Cancer Institute, the Health Insurance Plan (HIP) initiated a study of the efficacy of routinely scanning the breast for cancer back in the early 1960s. The subjects in the study were subjected to a physical examination of the breast and three additional exams, including mammography, each year for the period of the study (early 1960s to early 1970s). What the ten-year long HIP study showed was that clinical examination of the breast, coupled with routine mammography, can reduce the projected death rate of breast cancer by up to 30 percent.

A later study, dubbed the Breast Cancer Detection Demonstration Project (BCDDP), included a wide sample of women (250,000) aged 35 to 74 years. This nationwide study was implemented in 1973, again under the sponsorship of the NCI. A total of twenty-seven cancer screening centers were required to complete the full cycle of five annual screenings using physical palpation and examination of the breast, plus mammography, and thermography on each of the women.

Because of the justifiable concern over subjecting the women to high radiation exposure during screening, every effort was made to reduce exposure to the absolute minimum. One important advancement came out of this study. The scientists determined that it was possible to reduce the radiation dose to the breast midline well below 1 rad per exam without reducing the effectiveness of the screening. Thanks to these improved screening procedures, more and more patients and physicians alike are welcoming this method of detecting a small malignancy which is easy to surgically remove.

However, the experts say that methods for preventing the occurrence of breast cancer are far from clear while emphasizing the absolute necessity of early detection. Many of us are paying attention. A 1979 survey of women aged 20 to 64 years of age revealed that 63 percent had had a breast examination by a doctor within the past year, and another 20 percent said they had had such an examination within the past two years. By far,most women said that their physician had suggested the examination. One negative finding came out of this survey, however. Only one woman out of five reported having had a mammogram.

Cervical Cancer — Although the effectiveness of the Pap test has been questioned for a number of years, health specialists agree that this is a useful early detection procedure against cancer of the cervix. Most physicians routinely take a Pap smear during a physical examination. In other words, if you're a woman and go to the doctor for just about any reason, one of the questions you can expect is, "How long has it been since you had a Pap test?"

Surveys show that more than 70 percent of the women tallied had a Pap smear test regularly. Of this 70 percent, close to 60 percent reported having had a Pap test during the twelve months prior to the survey and another 20 percent reported having had the test within twenty-four months of the survey.

Overall, the death rate from cervical cancer has gone down slightly in recent years, but it can't be classified as a low risk. Especially at risk are the economically disadvantaged groups not covered by health care plans. For these people, routine physical examinations which include a Pap smear test (and breast examination) are not a reality of life. Without early detection, cancer of the cervix still kills.

Colorectal Cancer — For the population as a whole, the early detection of cancer of the colon or rectum just doesn't happen. Not enough doctors employ the use of the proctoscope to peer into the rectum, and few patients want to undergo this unpopular procedure. However, it must be pointed out that oncologists (cancer specialists) uniformly agree that a proctoscopic examination is the surest way to detect the early development of colorectal cancers. The experts say that once proctoscopy becomes a routine part of a general physical exam, we can look for a substantial reduction in the death rate of this type of cancer.

DO YOUR PART

Detecting a mass of cancerous (or precancerous) cells in its earliest stage gives you the best chance to beat it. Cancers which have not progressed to the stage where they produce noticeable symptoms are usually small, localized, and easily removed.

The American Cancer Society says that all of us should be intimately familiar with our bodies. Women are directed to examine their breasts monthly and be on the alert for lumps, a new thickening in the tissue, or any other change. Men are advised to be aware of the normal size and consistency of their testicles and to check them monthly for any change in the contour, an enlargement, or a difference in the degree of hardness.

The *Seven Warning Signals* of cancer are probably familiar to most of us, but they bear repeating. Watch out for:

1. Unusual bleeding or discharge.

2. A lump or thickening (breast or elsewhere).

3. A sore that does not heal.

4. A change in bowel or bladder habits.

5. A persistent cough or hoarseness.

6. Difficulty in swallowing or continual indigestion.

7. A change in a wart or mole.

Although the occurrence of any of these symptoms does not

necessarily mean you have cancer, the American Cancer Society recommends that you see your doctor immediately if any of these warning signals lasts longer than two weeks.

REGULAR PHYSICAL EXAM — A regular and thorough physical examination can be very useful in detecting even an early and symptomless malignancy. Your physican should conduct a detailed visual examination and palpitation of your entire body. His trained eyes and hands can spot an abnormality that might escape your notice. He will pay special attention to all body cavities, including the mouth, vagina, bladder (urogenital area), and rectum.

For some reason, all of us seem to reject the idea of a *proctosigmoidoscopy,* the examination of the rectum with a lighted tube. This simple and painless ten-minute procedure, albeit a little undignified, is extremely important in the early detection (and cure) of *colorectal* cancer, a malignant tumor of the colon or rectum. This type of examination is especially important for males because it will often show any prostate involvement as well.

Statistics show that the current death rate of women suffering from cervical cancer could be reduced by up to 90 percent if a yearly vaginal smear test (PAP) was a part of a regular physical examination. All women over 50 years of age are advised to have a soft-tissue x-ray (mammogram) of the breasts as well. Authorities say that, beginning at age 30, young women with a family history of breast cancer should have a baseline mammogram at least every other year.

ADDITIONAL DIAGNOSTIC PROCEDURES — *X-rays,* including the newer *CAT* scan (computer-aided tomography) which provides a more detailed visualization of internal masses than the original type of x-rays, give the physician a peek at what's going on internally. *Ultrasound,* high-frequency sound waves, registers differences in tissue and organ density and can show any abnormal changes which might be occurring.

A wide variety of *biochemical laboratory tests* on urine and blood can be useful in detecting specific cancers and are also used to monitor the effectiveness of treatment. *Cytology,* the microscopic examination of cell smears (taken from the mucous membranes of the nose, mouth, stomach and saliva) is a common early diagnostic procedure, but the results are considered inconclusive.

Most physicians prefer to follow up with an actual *biopsy* before diagnosing cancer. In a biopsy, a small piece of suspect tissue is surgically removed, stained, and viewed under a microscope for any tell-tale abnormalities. When indications of a possible cancer are strong, very often an anesthetized patient is kept on the table in the operating room while the tissue is being examined. This allows the physician to surgically remove the mass if laboratory tests confirm the presence of malignancy.

A *pathological* diagnosis of cancer is dependent on both the appearance of the biopsied tissue sample under a high-powered electron microscope and the clinical outcome of the case. In this type of procedure, the biochemical characteristics of the cells are critical and must be precisely evaluated by an expert laboratory pathologist.

In most instances, the management of a cancer patient's care and treatment is handled by an expert group of specialists, including a medical oncologist, surgeon, radiotherapist, and pathologist. These authorities consult with one another and minutely examine the details of the case to determine the best way to proceed.

TREATMENT: A LIMITED ARSENAL

SURGERY — The most effective way to eliminate cancer is to simply remove it surgically, along with neighboring tissue which may be suspect. When surgery is used in combination with advanced techniques employing radiation and chemotherapy, medical science has found that it is not really necessary to amputate an entire limb or breast to eradicate the cancer. The medical procedures available to the cancer specialist today have vastly improved in just the past five years alone.

In fact, you might want to spare a moment or two to be thankful that you are living in the modern world. It was not until the 19th century, when anesthesia and the benefit of antiseptic conditions were discovered, that surgery became a relatively safe and viable option for patients of the day. Further medical advances in the 20th century included immense improvements in surgical techniques, the introduction of blood transfusions, and powerful antibiotics to control infection.

Today, heart-lung pumps, artificial kidneys, the replacement of bones and blood vessels, plus the transplant of entire organs, seem almost commonplace. With these important further advances, suddenly all parts of the body have become accessible to the surgeon's knife.

SURGERY
Surgery to remove a tumor and nearby tissue remains the most effective way to cure many cancers. With radiation and chemotherapy, fewer amputations of limbs and breasts are performed than once were.

Although even more scientific and medical advances are coming slowly, surgically removing (excising) a cancerous mass completely is currently considered the optimum method of eliminating a malignancy. And it is, provided the tumor is enclosed and has not metastasized (spread) to other areas of the body.

From the time of Hippocrates, the abiding principle of medicine has always been *primum non nocere,* meaning "first, do no harm." Any surgeon worth his salt knows that there is an additional risk involved in 'opening up' any patient, particularly a cancer victim. If it is impossible to completely remove the malignancy, surgery can speed up the spread of cancer cells and actually shorten the life of the patient.

However, even when it is known in advance that a widespread cancer involving vital organs cannot be completely cut out, a surgeon can relieve the agonizing pain that is characteristic of some malignancies by severing critical nerve pathways. In addition, surgery may be necessary to relieve an internal obstruction or remove an abscess arising from either infection or the tumor itself.

As a valuable preventive measure, the physician may advise surgical removal of precancerous polyps in the colon or rectum, nodules in the thyroid gland, the uterus, certain pigmented moles, chronic ulcers, and some precancerous conditions arising inside the mouth.

Twenty years ago, a woman with a suspect lump in her breast often went into the operating room without knowing for certain whether she would undergo a complete *mastectomy* (surgical removal of the breast and neighboring nerves, muscles, lymph nodes, and tissue). If the waiting pathologist determined that her biopsied tissue was cancerous, the surgeon completely cut away the breast in an honest attempt to insure that all malignancy was eliminated.

Today, many women are considered candidates for a less disfiguring *lumpectomy,* in which merely the cancerous tumor and a small amount of surrounding tissue is removed. The good news is that a recent federally funded study of 1,843 breast-cancer patients shows that the five-year survival rate was 85 percent for women undergoing a lumpectomy in contrast to a 76 percent survival rate for women who had the complete mastectomy. In lumpectomy patients who were subsequently given radiation treatment, only 7.7 percent developed a recurring tumor in the same breast as opposed to 27.9 percent of those who had the lumpectomy only.

Women who must undergo a complete mastectomy because of extensive involvement will be glad to learn that breast reconstruction is becoming more and more common. The surgeon can save the nipple and sufficient skin, insert a prosthesis to match the natural breast, and then re-position the nipple in its normal place. Because the nerves have been cut, the nipple will no longer be sensitive to touch, but the appearance of the reconstructed breast is completely natural.

RADIATION THERAPY — In 1895, Wilhelm Roentgen discovered that electromagnetic rays had a rare power to penetrate animal tissue and give a picture of the internal workings of the body. Dubbed x-rays, this procedure was immediately acclaimed as an important diagnostic aid. It was not until 1910 that science determined that x-rays could lead to the development of cancer. But, on the other hand, skin cancers exposed to x-rays (or radium) disappeared. Now we come to the heart of the problem; how much exposure is valuable (and an acceptable risk in continuing to use x-rays in diagnosis and treatment) and how much is too much?

Radiotherapy treatment uses a source of ionizing radiation, such as x-rays, radium, or radioactive cobalt, for the destruction of malignant cancer cells. The trick is to bombard the complete cancerous mass (and any extensions or off-shoots) with radiation at the precise application which will destroy the tumor, but only cause minimal damage to normal tissue. The aim is to allow normal tissue to recover and survive the bombardment.

RADIATION THERAPY
Computerized controls, better methods of pinpointing the tumor, and new forms of radiation allow more selective destruction of tumors while sparing normal tissue. Chemicals are being tested to heighten a cancer's sensitivity to radiation.

With the development of multimillion volt equipment, high-speed delivery accomplishes a deeper and more sure penetration of tissue, more precise and sharper delineation of the field under attack, and less involvement of the neighboring normal tissue. Even newer types of sub-atomic particles (protons, neutrons, helium ions, pions) are being investigated for possible ways with which to increase the beneficial effects and broaden the range of this type of treatment.

Certain tumors (of the pancreas, stomach, esophagus, head, neck) have a strong resistance to conventional radiation therapy and some cancers are judged inoperable because they have invaded vital organs. It is these types of malignancies that science hopes will prove vulnerable to the more versatile forms of radiation. The results are encouraging and many researchers are expressing a guarded optimism.

Radiation is commonly used before a scheduled surgery to shrink the tumor to a more operable size. A new procedure, tested on more than 400 patients at U.S. cancer centers, involves bombarding the tumor directly with a massive dose of radiation during surgery while the patient is on the operating table. By directly targeting the area, there is no covering tissue in the way to sustain damage and very little involvement of neighboring tissue. The NCI cautions that it's too soon to evaluate long-term results in comparison with orthodox radiation therapy.

The aim of the radiologist is always to protect normal tissue while delivering a lethal dose of radiation to every malignant cell in a cancerous tumor. Another method of direct delivery being tested is the implant of a radioactive pellet into the tumor itself. Several types of malignancies, including breast cancer and prostatic cancer, are possible candidates for this type of treatment. The dose of radiation delivered to the tumor is maximized, while little can spill over into normal tissue.

NEUTRONS — According to data coming from the University of Washington (Seattle, Washington), neutrons (non-electric sub-atomic particles) have been used in the treatment of over 6000 patients, both here in the U.S. and abroad. Statistics appear to indicate that neutron radiation offers a strong advantage in the management of salivary gland tumors and prostatic cancer, but a only a slight advantage against bone, cartilege, and soft tissue malignancies.

PIONS — Pions or pi mesons (electrically charged particles of mass sized midway between electrons and protons) are being used in extensive medical trials at the Los Alamos National Laboratory (New Mexico). In 20 male patients suffering from prostatic cancer treated solely with pions, local control was achieved in 18. However, these very encouraging results were offset by the fact that only two patients out of a total of 59 victims of brain tumors (malignant glioma) responded favorably to pion irradiation.

Medical scientists in Switzerland experimenting with pion treatment report that this method has an excellent future against bladder cancer. In a group of 55 bladder cancer patients, the Swiss claim a complete response in 19 with total local control of the malignancy.

PROTONS — The Harvard Cyclotron Laboratory (Cambridge, Massachusetts) currently supplies four different hospitals and health-care facilities with protons (charged atomic particles) for their respective cancer treatment centers. Over the past decade, 965 patients have been irradiated with proton beams. Almost 600 of this group were being treated for a cancer in the back of the eyeball (choroidal melanoma), notoriously difficult to eliminate or control without complete removal of the eyeball itself. The proton treatment chalked up an astounding local control rate of 98 percent.

In a group of 67 patients with a rare form of cancer (chordoma or chondrosarcoma: tumor formed at the base of the skull or spine), the local control rate was a very satisfactory 89 percent of those treated with proton beams. This figure was confirmed and locked in more than a year after treatment during a follow-up evaluation of each patient.

Unfortunately, those being treated with protons for an inoperable brain tumor (glioma) did not fare so well. Of the seven patients thus treated, only one can be considered a long-term survivor. The other six died within a few months of completing treatment.

HELIUM IONS — The University of California (San Francisco, California) has also reported success against spinal cord tumors (chondrosarcomas) and eye tumors (choroidal melanonomas). Using helium ions (a combination of two protons and two neutons), these medical scientists have treated 190 patients suffering with a tumor behind the eyeball and

45

report achieving local control in 116. A total of 27 of the group developed cataracts, making cataracts a significant complication of treatment. Inasmuch as cataract surgery is routinely performed today, that would seem to be a fair tradeoff.

Although the California researchers have treated only 19 patients with cancerous spinal cord involvement, local control was achieved in 15. Control has been documented in follow-up evaluations ranging from two months to over two years in some of the cases.

Working against time, as did the physicians of previous centuries, the radiologists of our time are now involved in an intensive evaluation of the different sources of ionizing radiation and are attempting to work out the filtration, distance factors, and sequence of doses best used against the wide variety of cancers that respond poorly to conventional radiation and other forms of treatment.

CHEMOTHERAPY
Scientists are working to limit the side effects of chemotherapy. Some are searching for new toxic agents to kill cancer cells, while others are synthesizing less toxic cousins of existing drugs. Combinations of drugs have proved more effective than single-drug treatments.

CHEMOTHERAPY — At its most optimistic and hopeful, *chemotherapy* is defined as "the application of chemical reagents which are not harmful to the patient, but which have a specific and toxic effect on disease-causing micro-organisms." (Taber's Cyclopedic Medical Dictionary). Unfortunately, we've all heard horror stories of the debilitating and sometimes agonizing side-effects of chemotherapy.

However, this is not to imply that chemotherapy is a treatment to be avoided at all costs. Certain cancers respond very favorably to this treatment, including *choriocarcinoma* (tumor originating in the placenta), and *Burkitt's lymphoma* (tumor of the lymph system). The cure rate of chemotherapy against these two particularly malignant forms of cancer is very high. Children suffering from acute *leukemia* (blood cancer) treated with a combination of chemotherapy drugs often enjoy long-term periods of disease-free remission, as do patients in even the most advanced stages of *Hodgkin's disease,* which affects the spleen, liver, and lymphoid tissue.

In an attempt to overcome one of the most debilitating effects of some chemotherapy drugs, scientists are testing new anti-nausea agents to prevent the uncontrolled vomiting and severe nausea that causes some patients to refuse treatment. Showing great promise as a nausea preventive is *nabilone,* one of the effective ingredients in marijuana. When nabilone is given before chemotherapy begins, nausea can be reduced to bearable proportions.

One of the problems faced by medical science is the fact that most cancer drugs have a limited usefulness. In a tumor, only a certain percentage of the malignant cells are dividing at any given time. Most drugs can effectively destroy only the part of the cells undergoing division. Some cancer cells develop a resistance to the drugs and render them ineffective. An even greater problem is the fact that tumor cells require such a large amount of a drug to destroy them that normal cells are destroyed as well.

In order to overcome these effects, combinations of chemo-therapeutic agents which act on cells in different ways are used in various treatment programs, either simultaneously or in a measured sequence. By combining or varying the drugs used, there is less irreparable damage to normal cells and the tendency of malignant cells to become resistant to a single agent is counteracted.

COMBINING DRUGS — The National Cancer Institute reports that encouraging results are attained with the com-bination of *adriamycin,* a common anticancer chemotherapeutic agent, and *verapamil.* Verapamil is a drug used to control heart *arrhythmias* (irregular heartbeat). NCI researchers say that the evidence gathered thus far indicates that the addition of verapamil can counter the ability of some cancer cells to resist chemotherapy.

Although it is known to destroy kidney cells, *cisplatin* is nevertheless a valuable and widely used chemotherapy drug. Scientists have determined that when the patient is infused with a saline (salt) solution along with cisplatin, the salt renders the cisplatin less toxic to kidney cells, giving the drug time to attack the cancer.

The cisplatin/saline combination proved beneficial in women with ovarian cancer and men with third-stage (advanced) cancer of the testicles. With a projected cure rate of only 50 percent by the usual treatment, the cure rate of men given this combination therapy jumped to a very encouraging 85 to 90 percent.

However, given the protective effect exerted on the kidney cells by the saline solution, another problem surfaced. Cisplatin is also highly toxic to nerve cells. The NCI is now working to find a way to counteract this additional barrier to the use of cisplatin.

CIRCADIAN TIMING — Another factor under study is the circadian timing of drug administration. In dissecting this term, we find *circa* (about) *dian* (day) refers to the fact that certain biological rhythms of the body are known to occur approximately every 24 hours. Studies have shown that simply taking these internal biological changes into account and timing the administration of adriamycin and cisplatin accordingly has a profound effect on the body's ability to handle the toxicity of the drugs.

A paper issued by the University of Minnesota Medical School and the Masonic Cancer Center (Minneapolis, Minnesota) says that "The most crucial element in the successful application of cancer chemotherapy is optimization of the effects and minimization of toxicity to normal tissue. One approach to increasing this selectivity is administration of these highly toxic drugs at times associated with best tolerance."

In a study of the effects of cherotherapy on 31 patients suffering with advanced ovarian cancer, the researchers found that the administration of *adriamycin in the morning* and *cisplatin in the evening* was more easily tolerated and resulted in far fewer side effects and consequent interruption of treatment. For instance, in the control group receiving the drugs in the reverse order, drug dosages had to be modified downward three times as often, complications and side effects were doubled, and four times as many treatments had to be delayed while the patient regained the strength to continue.

DRUGS DISGUISED — In another attempt to lessen the toxicity of chemotherapy agents to normal cell tissue, both the University of North Carolina Medical School (Chapel Hill, North Carolina) and the University of Illinois (Urbana, Illinois) have bound anticancer drugs, such as adriamycin, to the same type of protein that is found in a common blood clot. A drug in the guise of a blood clot doesn't bind as easily to normal cells. Cells in the area of a malignant tumor gobble up the protein, therby releasing the drug and activating it directly at the site of the cancer.

A spokesman for the University of North Carolina explains, "For most anticancer drugs, the difference between the toxic dose and the effective dose is pitifully small. By taking advantage of the biochemical differences between normal and malignant cells, we don't necessarily make the drugs more effective for fighting cancer, just less toxic to normal cells."

CANCER CONTROL

Preventing cancer from invading your body is the best defense, but controlling cancer by finding it early is an important and viable second line of defense available to us all. The National Cancer Institute is going all out on a strong program of education and is encouraging state health agencies and industry to implement their own risk assessment programs. Health maintenance organizations are springing up everywhere. At the end of 1985, over 400 HMOs with a combined membership of close to 20 million were functioning. For these 20 million people, regular physical examinations utilizing advanced cancer detection procedures are a reality. Efficient screening programs have been shown to be invaluable in the control of cancer.

IS THE KILLER WINNING? — As things stand right now, we appear to be willing to settle for a draw. Even with all its considerable forces mobilized and on the attack, medical science cannot say just when cancer will be conquered. To be sure, we are taking two giant steps forward in the fight against cancer for every one step backward. We are inching toward a better understanding of the various forms of the disease and trying new and more effective methods of treatment and therapy every year. The most brilliant scientific and medical minds in the world are working to find a solution to this condition which frightens even the most fearless among us, but . . .

PREVENTION REMAINS THE BEST SOLUTION — There are many natural and holistic ways with which you can help yourself. You must examine your lifestyle and make whatever changes necessary in order to protect yourself and your loved ones from the spectre stalking us all. You can be a victor and not a victim. We can point the way, but only you can make the right choices.

Nutritional & Holistic Treatments
Ways You Can Help Yourself

Chapter IV
Diet, Nutrition, Cancer & More
Science Finally Recognizes That "We Are What We Eat"

A few years ago, a special committee of the National Research Council was appointed by the National Academy of Sciences to find out if what we eat (or don't eat) has anything to do with the development of cancer. The committee was chaired by Dr. Clifford Grobstein of the University of California and included fourteen highly respected scientists. The committee studied and evaluated thousands of research papers conducted by hundreds of other scientists. The final report, entitled *Diet, Nutrition, and Cancer*, was published in 1982.

You might be pardoned for thinking that everyone in the U.S. immediately ransacked their homes and pitched out all the foods the committee discovered which *increase* the risk of developing cancer. You might think it's only logical that grocery shoppers everywhere began shopping more selectively to choose foods which the council reports will *reduce* the risk of developing cancer. This information is so valuable to life and health that you might expect that a large percentage of the population promptly took whatever steps were necessary and changed their diet to conform with these important dietary guidelines.

But that's not what happened. The American Cancer Society, the National Cancer Institute and the Government Printing Office all prepared attractive, easy-to-understand *free* brochures with the dietary guidelines clearly laid out. Television and radio gave the report full coverage. Newspapers, magazines, and even books headlined the findings of the committee. After all the hoopla, it's hard to believe that there's anyone in these United States who hasn't been exposed to this information in some form or other. The general public received the good news with a big 'ho-hum.'

It's time and past time to pay attention. In fact, for some, it may be almost too late. Even though you can't change or control *all* the risk factors that combine to determine how susceptible you are to cancer a family health history which shows an hereditary tendency toward the disease, for instance (See Chapter 11.) — you can certainly change and control every mouthful of food you swallow every day.

Science now recognizes that dietary factors play a major part in the development of cancer. As long ago as the early 1940s, researchers observed that diet influenced the progress of cancer. In laboratory animals with chemically-induced carcinogenic tumors, a high calorie and/or a high fat diet caused the tumors to grow at a rapid rate. The Committee on Diet, Nutrition, and Cancer (Assembly of Life Sciences, National Research Council, National Academy Press, Washington, D.C., 1982) has stressed the relationship between dietary fat intake and the incidence of various cancers. Dietary fat not only promotes harmful high blood fat levels, but also affects our immune response by inhibiting the action of important components (lymphocytes, macrophages) of the immune system.

Now that we know about the preventive effect eating the right foods can offer against cancer (and the other killing degenerative diseases), it is of primary importance that we review the factors that science says can *increase* or *decrease our risk of developing this dread disease.*

FACTORS INCREASING THE RISK OF CANCER:

- Fats (saturated/chemically-altered)
- Cholesterol
- Intake of total calories
- Dietary Proteins (meats)
- Carcinogenic Chemicals in Food
  - Processing
  - Storage
  - Preparation
  - Packaging
- Nitrosamines
- Smoked Foods
- Pesticides/Herbicides (agricultural chemicals)
- Coffee & Tea
- Tobacco

FACTORS DECREASING THE RISK OF CANCER

- Vitamins
  - Vitamin A (retinoids)
  - Beta-Carotene (provitamin A)
  - Vitamin C (ascorbic acid)
  - Vitamin E (d-tocopherol)
  - Vitamin B2 (riboflavin)
- Minerals
  - Selenium
  - Zinc
- Dietary Fiber
- Vegetables

An involved and detailed investigation of cancer rates and eating habits in the United States as compared to a number of other countries around the world strongly suggests that cancer can be markedly reduced simply by making some sensible changes in the way we eat and live. Authorities believe the incidence of colon cancer and breast cancer, in particular, can be brought down. As these stand now in the U.S., 50,000 of us die of colon cancer every year, and breast cancer claims 40,000 American women every year. In cancer-related deaths, colon and breast tumors are exceeded only by lung cancer, which currently accounts for 120,000 victims every year in this country. The American Cancer Society estimates that diet plays a crucial part in at least 35 percent of all cancer cases in the U.S. After you finish reading this book, I think you'll agree with me that the percentage is really a lot higher. The National Research Council's findings, in brief, as published by The American Cancer Society follow.

PREVENTIVE NUTRITION

CRUCIFEROUS VEGETABLES — According to recent research, the cabbage-family vegetables exert a protective effect against respiratory system cancers, stomach cancers, and colorectal (colon and rectal) cancers. The cruciferous vegetables, so named for their cross-shaped flowers, include all types of cabbages, broccoli, cauliflower, brussels sprouts and kale.

Just what is it in these vegetables that's responsible for their protective effect? The cabbage family cousins all contain special compounds called *indoles.* Tests on laboratory animals show that feeding animals certain indoles before introducing cancer-causing substances can prevent the expected malignancies from forming.

Researchers know that putting the carcinogen *BaP* (benzo[a]pyrene) in the upper esophagus of mice will bring on stomach cancer. Another carcinogen known as *DMBA* (7,12-dimethylbenz[a]anthracene) will cause breast cancers when fed to rats. Both these methods are commonly used in laboratory studies to develop cancer in test animals. In exhaustive experiments, the animals fed indoles before the introduction of the chemical carcinogens remained free of tumors, but the control group of animals not protected by indoles in their food developed malignant cancers right on schedule.

The experts say that including cabbage-family vegetables in the diet will supply the natural indoles that provide such strong anti-cancer protection.

HIGH-FIBER — Publishing in the *Southern Medical Journal,* David M. Vanderpool, B.S., Texas Tech University School of Medicine (Lubbock, Texas), notes that during the past century, the role of the indigestible constituents of food, such as fiber, have been overlooked. Dr. Vanderpool says, "With the advent of milling, the bran and germ of cereal grains were removed, e sugar of cane was pressed out and crystallized, and the oil was taken from seeds. The result of these processes was a revolution in the dietary formula of the civilized world. More than half of the calories in our everyday diet now come from refined foods that contain little or no indigestible fiber."

Dr. Vanderpool points out that it has been known since the time of Socrates (469-399 BC) that consuming high-fiber foods increases daily stool weight. Studies show that the usual diet of the civilized world, lacking in fiber, produces stool weights of about 100 grams, but African natives eating high-fiber foods have normal stools of 500 grams. Our consumption of refined foods has led to a steadily increasing incidence of appendicitis, diverticular disease, duodenal ulcer disease — and cancer of the colon.

Dr. Vanderpool says, "Epidemiologists indicate that carcinoma of the colon is a result of industrialization. During this century, the western world has experienced a dramatic increase in the incidence of carcinoma of the colon, which has paralleled the decrease in dietary fiber intake. As animal proteins and saturated fats have supplanted cereal grains and tuberous carbohydrates, colon cancer has become more common. With decreased fiber, fecal bulk is reduced, increasing the concentration of carcinogens. In addition, decreased motility of the colon allows the carcinogenic material to stay in the colon for longer period."

The high-fiber foods offer particularly strong protection against colon cancer. Foods which are high in fiber include all whole grains, nuts, fruits, and vegetables. Add more fiber to your daily diet with whole-grain cereals (one bowl of All-Bran provides 10 grams) and breads (120 grams of whole wheat provides another 10 grams), potatoes, rice, spinach, fruits, tomatoes, and even popcorn. All of the legumes, such as peas and beans (lentils, soybeans, kidney beans, limas, black beans), are a good source of healthy fiber, as is corn.

Research indicates that most of us need from four-times to *ten-times* as much fiber as we consume daily. In order to work efficiently, the body requires about 40 grams of fiber daily, but the average diet of today's refined, denatured and processed foods provides only a fraction of that amount — about 4 grams. Dr. Vanderpool emphasizes, "If one accepts 40 grams of fiber per day as an adequate goal for reducing the risk of colonic disease, only minimal modification of the diet would be necessary to reach that goal."

Fiber keeps the entire gastro-intestinal tract running smoothly. In fact, a very welcome side-effect of the high-fiber diet is the fact that constipation will never be a problem. Although fiber will certainly correct constipation, it is not a 'laxative.' Fiber moves food through the body efficiently without the harmful 'blast out' effect of chemical laxatives which interrupt the normal functioning of the bowels.

As a cancer-preventive, a study conducted at the Virginia Polytechnic Institute by Dr. Tracy Wilkins determined that certain bacteria normally present in the bowel die and produce a potent carcinogen called *fecapentaene*. However, when a fiber-rich diet is ingested, the bacteria remains healthy. In the presence of fiber in the intestinal tract, the bacteria doesn't die and therefore doesn't release harmful fecapentaene.

Increasing the intake of fiber also increases the growth of friendly intestinal bacteria available to process our food *and* fiber aids in retaining the important B vitamins. Studies have shown that valuable organisms are drastically decreased on a so-called 'smooth' diet low in fiber and some individuals deficient in fiber actually harbor certain intestinal bacteria which produce a B-complex destroying enzyme.

Also under study are the effects of the ratio of *fiber to fat* in the diet. Examining the facts, we find that the Japanese people traditionally have a very low incidence of colon cancer, but generally eat the same amount of high fiber foods as Americans. Studies show that the main difference in the eating habits of the peoples of the two nations is that the typical Japanese diet contains only about half the fat of the typical U.S. diet. Early conclusions suggest that a low-fat diet coupled with a high-fiber diet provides the most protection against possible cancer development.

VITAMIN A — Deep orange fruits and vegetables provide an abundance of beta-carotene, which the body uses to manufacture Vitamin A. Carrots, peaches, apricots and squash all qualify, as does broccoli, and are best consumed fresh. Studies show that beta-carotene protects against cancers of the larynx, lungs, and esophagus.

A British researcher, Richard Peto of Oxford, England, has been quoted as saying that there's a very strong possibility that beta-carotene could prevent up to one-third of the cancer deaths in the U.S. because it acts to protect the genetic programming in each cell from possible damage by free radicals. Science has shown that free radicals, a by-product of fat metabolism, can turn a healthy cell into a malignant one.

The American Cancer Society has announced that fresh foods are a better source of Vitamin A than vitamin pills. The main dietary sources of Vitamin A itself (the retinoids) are the organ meats (liver, in particular), milk and cheese. You should, of course, select low-fat dairy products to avoid ingesting too much fat.

The ACS warns against the use of Vitamin A supplements, which can be toxic in excessive amounts. Unless your doctor has determined that you are deficient in Vitamin A and prescribed the proper daily dose for you, it's best to depend on good nutrition for your supply of this important vitamin. Doses of over 50,000 I.U. (International Units) per day can be dangerous.

On the other hand, beta-carotene has no known toxicity and no apparent upper limits of ingestion. The only thing that happens if you overdose on foods rich in beta-carotene is that your skin will take on a yellow tinge.

Interestingly enough, some solid studies on beta-carotene and Vitamin A have been conducted in various areas of the world almost simultaneously in recent times. The College of Medicine in New York discovered that women with a low beta-carotene/Vitamin A intake were subject to a much greater risk (three times) of developing either a precancerous condition known as *cervical dysplasia* and cervical cancer itself than the control group.

In Milan, Italy, an investigative body of doctors came up with the same conclusions. The Italians determined that women whose average intake of beta-carotene topped 5,000 I.U. daily had a significantly less risk of contracting cervical cancer. The Italian study found that women ingesting only Vitamin A, but not beta-carotene, did not receive the same protection.

A 20-year ongoing study still in progress in Japan found that individuals eating beta-carotene foods regularly have a lower risk of developing lung, stomach, and other cancers. The researchers determined that there was over a 25 percent reduction in stomach cancers in those who simply increased their daily vegetable consumption.

The British Columbia Cancer Research Center in Vancouver conducted a rigidly-controlled study with a group of quid-chewing Filipinos living in rural Luzon, the Philippines. Quid-chewing, an ancient practice, accounts for hundreds of thousands of oral cancer deaths in Asia every year. The quid is prepared with the betal leaf, the areca nut, dried tobacco leaves, and roasted snail shells. The snail shells are roasted and crushed to a powder, adding a strong lime content to the quid. The Filipinos used in the study commonly chewed from four to fifteen quids daily.

Medical volunteers provided their subjects with 100,000 I.U. of Vitamin A daily and 300,000 I.U. of beta-carotene was administered weekly. The three-month study was so short that the researchers were aware there was little chance of cancer developing. Instead, they probed for cell damage in the mucous membranes of the mouth, a warning sign of early malignancy. At the beginning of the study, the tissue samples showed many damaged cells. At the conclusion of the study, the same subjects showed a dramatic decrease in the number of damaged cells, although all had continued to chew their cancer-promoting quids. The researchers documented a 40 percent decrease in the number of damaged cells each month the study continued.

This important Canadian research shows that dietary changes may act to save us from the harmful effects of ingrained bad habits. According to Dr. Eli Seifter of the Albert Einstein College of Medicine in New York, rats given beta-carotene more than thirty days after exposure to a carcinogenic chemical did not develop the expected tumors. Dr. Seifter says, "Even after exposure to cancer-producing doses of toxic chemicals, beta-carotene still has its effect. Beta-carotene is protective against either late stage tumor development or the early stages of tumor growth."

Dr. Seifter says his research suggests that a daily intake of 5 to 10 milligrams of beta-carotene provides protection against certain tumors. The doctor says that high risks, such as smokers, will require twice that amount.

When mother said, "Eat your carrots, dear; they're good for you," she didn't know how very right she was!

VITAMIN C — You probably already know that most fruits, including grapefruit, cantaloupes, oranges, and strawberries, are an excellent source of Vitamin C. Red and green bell peppers, tomatoes, and broccoli also qualify. Vitamin C is considered strong protection against cancers of the stomach and esophagus, possibly because it has the ability to prevent the body from manufacturing cancer-causing nitrosamines from some chemically cured foods. (see *Nitrosamines* this chapter.)

As a treatment for cancer, Vitamin C is showing astounding properties. A practicing oncologist in Fukuoka, Japan, Fukumi Morishige, M.D., Ph.D., and his associates have been regularly treating both terminal and seriously diseased cancer patients with Vitamin C for over thirty years. Dr. Morishige has published data indicating that large doses of Vitamin C can increase the life expectancy of even terminal cancer patients.

Even more exciting is the news that a mixture of Vitamin C and copper appears to be a cancer-killer of incredible potential. Laboratory mice, cancer infested and close to dying, treated with this mixture had their lifespan increased beyond previously known limits.

The doctor reports on the case of a woman in her mid-thirties suffering terribly from incurable bone cancer (osteosarcoma) which was untouched by chemotherapy. Her left arm was paralyzed and the pain she endured could not be relieved by even the strongest painkillers. She was doomed to die an agonizing death until she was given regular injections of megadoses of Vitamin C and the copper compound.

Dr. Morishige's report states, "Two months' treatment relieved the intolerable pain and paralysis of the diseased left arm. From x-ray examinations, the tumor lesion was found to have completely disappeared after four months of this treatment." Two years after she was released, this fortunate woman is still free of cancer.

In spite of the good results researchers around the world have received with Vitamin C therapy, including the study published in 1976 by the renowned Nobel laureate Linus Pauling, Ph.D. and Ewan Cameron, M.D.,indicating that megadoses of Vitamin C actually extend the lifespan of terminal cancer victims, the controversy over the benefits of Vitamin C continues. The results of the Mayo Clinic study as published in the New England Journal of Medicine (January 1985) were disappointing. The Mayo Clinic report concludes that high-dose Vitamin C therapy is not effective against advanced cancer.

Dr. Pauling rebuts that statement with the following comments. "Mayo clinic patients received Vitamin C for just a short time, an average of only 2½ *months*. None of the Mayo Clinic patients died while taking Vitamin C, but these patients did die after they were taken off Vitamin C. Our patients received high doses of Vitamin C until time of death — for as long as *12 years* in some cases!'

VITAMIN D & CALCIUM — Although the American Cancer Society report does not specifically target Vitamin D as a cancer-preventive nutrient, there's enough evidence around to suggest that this vitamin may play an important part. A report authored by Cedric Garland of the University of California at San Diego, School of Medicine, indicates that persons who include Vitamin D and high calcium foods regularly in their diet have one-third the rate of colorectal cancer as others who seldom ingest such foods.

Using data collected over a period of 19 years, Dr. Garland and his brother, Frank Garland of the Naval Health Research Center in San Diego, determined that in the group of 2000 men in the study, those who ingested low levels of both Vitamin D and calcium showed a colorectal cancer incidence of 38.9 per 1,000. On the other hand, the men who ate a diet rich in these important nutrients had a colorectal cancer rate of only 14.3 per 1,000.

An even earlier regional study on the effects of sunshine on health showed that people who live in southern and western states and who necessarily absorb a lot of natural sunshine, known to promote Vitamin D levels in the body, had a much lower incidence of colorectal cancer than the populations of northern and eastern states where the sun does not shine as strongly or as often. (Note: see *Sunshine* this chapter.)

VITAMIN E — Researchers at the University of Colorado recently determined that Vitamin E can stop the growth of pro-state cancer cells, at least in a test-tube. This information is hardly a surprise. Earlier laboratory studies confirm that Vitamin E can destroy malignant cells outright and/or inhibit their proliferation.

Vitamin E acts by stimulating the immune system and maintaining white blood cell and cell membrane configurations, necessary to normal functioning. Although not as powerful as some other antioxidants, Vitamin E protects against the DNA damaging free radicals which cause mutations and cancer. Antioxidants lessen the mutation rate considerably. It has been shown that laboratory animals deliberately injected with live cancer cells have a better chance to survive when given Vitamin

E at the rate of up to 2,000 I.U. for every kilogram of fodder. Vitamin E is used up rapidly by the body. It is important to note that Vitamin E must be ingested regularly and continually to provide protection.

SELENIUM — In the mid-1960s, both U.S. and Canadian researchers reported that in areas where the soil was rich in selenium, a powerful antioxidant, the human cancer death rates were lower than in areas where selenium levels were deficient. Laboratory studies appear to indicate that cancer rates can be reduced by up to 70 percent with selenium supplements. The National Cancer Institute believes that 200 micrograms daily of selenium (sodium selenite) should be included in the RDA (Recommended Daily Allowance) tables by the FDA.

However, a note of caution comes from the National Academy of Science regarding selenium supplements. Too much selenium can be toxic, especially in conjunction with low-protein ingestion. Until all the evidence is in, it would be wise to seek professional medical advice before making the decision to include selenium supplements in your cancer-preventive program.

EATING LESS — An important part of an effective preventive nutrition program is that of weight control. Studies have shown that obesity is a contributing factor in cancers of the uterus, gallbladder, breast and colon. Lowering your total caloric intake (and following the guidelines given above when shopping and planning meals) will greatly reduce your odds of contracting cancer. An exercise regime suited to the age and condition of the individual is very helpful in controlling weight.

Studies show a strong connection between obesity and cancer-prone individuals. Between 1960 and 1972, the ACS conducted a long-term study of 750,000 persons. The statistics gleaned from this research show very clearly that high rates of certain cancers are common among the obese. Obesity is usually clinically defined as those who are approximately 40 percent over the average standard weight for their frame size. The risk of developing cancer was tabulated as 55 percent higher than normal for obese women and 33 percent higher than normal for obese men.

Additional research shows that laboratory animals which are consistently underfed and deliberately kept lean and trim are less susceptible to the development of cancer and tumor growth. Animals on a high calorie diet do not appear to be so favored.

RISKY NUTRITION

FAT — It's easier than you might think to reduce your overall fat intake simply by making a few changes. Start by selecting lean cuts of meat. Remove the skin from chicken and other poultry before cooking and learn to love fish unbreaded, perhaps poached in a little court bullion (fish stock) for rich flavor. Use only low-fat dairy products and pass up pastries and other fat-loaded sweets. Another obvious benefit is that reducing fat in the diet helps keep weight down. A diet high in fat has been shown to increase the risk of breast, colon and prostate cancer.

Studies of various groups support this fact. For instance, the Japanese people traditionally eat a diet very low in fats in their homeland. But when they migrate to the U.S. and change their diet to correspond with western standards, their incidence of both breast and colon cancer rises dramatically. The death rate from cancer in America is five to ten times higher than in Japan.

Certain close-knit and health-conscious religious groups also exhibit a much lower incidence of cancer in general (and colon cancer in particular) than does the general population. The approximately 600,000 Seventh Day Adventists in the U.S. commonly eat a largely vegetarian diet which is also low in fats. A recent study showed that Seventh Day Adventists run a much lower risk of dying of colorectal cancers, smoke-related cancers, and breast cancer than a comparable group of nonmembers. The Mormons, although not strict vegetarians, follow a very healthy lifestyle. The use of tobacco, caffeinated beverages, and alcoholic spirits are forbidden. The Utah Cancer Registry has data which shows the incidence of lung, colorectal, breast, ovarian, and uterine cancer is far lower among Mormons than the national average. Interestingly, there is no difference in the incidence of prostate cancer in Mormon men than in the general population.

The scientists say that fat itself probably is not a primary cause of colon cancer, but instead nourishes the development of tumors caused by other substances. Fats increase the secretion of digestive juices (bile acids and steroids). It appears that the extra digestive chemicals needed to break down excessive fat intake may actually damage the walls of the intestines and thereby allow carcinogens to enter.

In breast cancer, a high fat diet contributes to obesity. The theory here is that carrying excess weight increases the body's production of the female hormone *estrogen,* which speeds up and fosters the growth of tumors.

An important fact to note in this context is that, as far as cancer development is concerned, it doesn't seem to matter what type of fat is consumed. Polyunsaturated fats are just as much a factor in cancer growth as are saturated fats, named by the American Heart Association as increasing the risk of heart disease because of their cholesterol content. Although the American Heart Association recommends polyunsaturates as preferable to saturated fats, both the American Cancer Society and the Heart Association are urging us to reduce our *total intake* of fats. The ACS says that only 30 percent of the day's calories should be consumed in fat. As things stand at this writing, the general public usually takes in more than 40 percent of the day's calories in fat. Both these prestigious agencies say that trimming away a mere 10 percent of fat from our daily meals will bring great benefits. (See Chapters 5 and 6.)

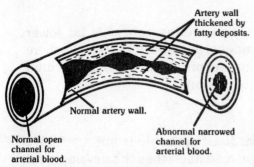

Artery wall thickened by fatty deposits.

Normal artery wall.

Normal open channel for arterial blood.

Abnormal narrowed channel for arterial blood.

  HEALTHY ARTERY

  EARLY LESION

 SMALL FAT DEPOSIT

 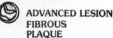 ADVANCED LESION FIBROUS PLAQUE

ADVANCED LESION CAUSING

HEART INFARCTION   STROKE   GANGRENE   ANEURYSM

Cross-Sections of Clogged Arteries

Blood flow
Atheroma
Blood clot

Atheroma formation

An atheroma, or patch of fatty tissue that damages arterial walls, tends to form at the point at which an artery branches and the flow of blood is naturally disturbed. As atheroma increases, atherosclerosis develops.

Roughened artery wall
Atheroma
Blood flow

CHOLESTEROL — Almost 30 percent of the nearly two million deaths in the U.S. each year are caused by coronary heart disease arising as a result of cholesterol-clogged arteries that supply the heart. Over time, the arteries narrow, the flow of blood is restricted, atherosclerosis develops, and a heart attack occurs. Cholesterol is present in all foods of animal origin and is part of every animal cell.

High serum cholesterol is one of the three major risk factors in coronary heart disease, but one you can control. (The other two risk factors, which are fortunately also controllable, are high blood pressure and cigarette smoking.) The experts say that the typical American diet, high in saturated fats, raises blood cholesterol levels. As serum cholesterol rises, the risk of suffering a heart attack keeps pace and we are at additional risk of developing certain forms of cancer as well.

Because the ingestion of cholesterol-producing saturated fats has been officially labeled as being of great harm to the body, this next statement may surprise you. *The body itself can manufacture cholesterol in quantities of about 1.5 grams daily.* Cholesterol is the material the body uses to produce bile acids, certain hormones and provitamin D3. If cholesterol in the diet is reduced, the body goes into production and increases its manufacture. Studies indicate that diets deliberately kept low in cholesterol are often ineffective in reducing serum cholesterol levels in the blood because cholesterol is a fat. Like all fats, cholesterol is insoluble in water or blood. In order to transport it, the body transforms it into a lipoprotein (a combination of fat and protein). The trick is to keep the cholesterol in a liquid state so that it isn't deposited on arterial walls. The body does this very nicely when it's provided with the high-density lipo-proteins (HDL) *lecithin* and *linoleic acid.* Interestingly enough, the very foods forbidden on a so-called low cholesterol diet (butter, milk, eggs, cheese, well-marbled beef), also contain more than enough HDL to keep cholesterol liquid and moving through the body.

The melting point of cholesterol itself is 300 degrees F. At the normal body temperature of 98.6 degrees, cholesterol ends up as a deposit on arterial walls, leading undeniably to atherosclerotic plaque. However, when lecithin, a saturated fatty acid, is supplied, the melting point of cholesterol comes down to 180 degrees, admittedly still insoluble at normal body temperature. But when a linoleate-containing dietary fat is supplied along with the lecithin, cholesterol liquifies at a cool 32 degrees F. These HDLs keep cholesterol liquid, the body absorbs what it needs, and no plaque accumulates on arterial walls to cause problems. Abracadabra! Why is it that some authorities think Mother Nature doesn't know what she's doing?

We are drifting a bit off center from our main subject of fats as they contribute to cancer, but you should know that a study of 900 men examined for signs of early atherosclerosis deter-mined that those with more than 36 percent HDL in their blood had no atherosclerosis, but those with 34 percent or less HDL had evidence of the disease.

COMMERCIALLY PROCESSED FATS — Let's take a quick look at the process that brings us vegetable oils and margarine.

Vegetable seeds are crushed to release their oils and then put through a solvent (carbon tetrachloride or methylene chloride) to leach out the last bit of marketable oil. The resulting mess is then boiled to evaporate off as much of the chemical solvent as possible.

The next step is to remove whatever natural fatty acids remain, usually somewhere around 6 percent. The oil is cooked at temperatures of approximately 150 degrees F. with a solution of lye, producing an elementary type of soap which settles to the bottom of the witch's cauldron (processing chamber). The lighter oil is skimmed off, but the manufacturers still aren't satisfied.

Any so-called 'impurities' which remain (including important nutrients such as lecithin and carotene, a precursor of Vitamin A) are either filtered out through the same kind of adsorbent earth you use to clean your swimming pool or removed chemically. Placed in a vacuum, the oil is heated yet again to temperatures ranging as high as 380 degrees F. and held at temperature for at least 12 hours to completely deodorize it.

If the end product is to be a margarine, the manufacturer further subjects the oils to the hydrogenation process which alters the melting point to mimic the hardness of butter. Finally, an antioxidant (usually butylated hydroxyanisole) is added to extend shelf-life and the product ends up in the supermarket looking very attractive indeed.

Because the calorie count of the fat is not changed by all this chemical processing, the manufacturer can label the product accordingly. Unfortunately, nutritional scientists seem unaware that the resulting *unnatural* polyunsaturates possess as yet unknown biological properties. The one thing that *is* certain is that no natural nutrients remain. (See Chapter 5 for a detailed report on these destructive fats.)

Note: Only linseed (flax), pumpkin, soy, and walnut oils contain both essential fatty acids (linoleic and linolenic). The experts caution that these oils must be the cold-pressed, unrefined, natural varieties, and not the processed abominations found in most supermarkets. (See Chapters 5 and 6.)

NITROSAMINES — The American Cancer Society has determined that cancers of the esophagus and stomach are common in areas of the world where smoked, salt-cured, and nitrite-cured meats are eaten in large quantities. Many Americans find ham, bacon, sausage and hot dogs irresistible. These foods contain chemicals (nitrosamines and PAHs, polycyclic aromatic hydrocarbons) which cause cancer in animals. To be on the safe side, The American Cancer Society recommends that these foods, as well as salt-cured and smoked fish, be eaten only occasionally.

Nitrosamines are produced in the body from nitrites and nitrates used in curing certain foods. As an important additive in processing, these chemicals prevent the formation of deadly botulism spores which can cause death when they occur in foods. Unfortunately, the nitrosamines the body manufactures from foods cured in this manner are extremely carcinogenic.

Since this fact has become increasingly clear, science has been attempting to find ways to reduce the risk. It has been shown that Vitamin C can help prevent the body from manufacturing cancer-causing nitrosamines from nitrites. The meat industry is cooperating by adding Vitamin C to many chemically-cured products and has lowered their nitrite content as well. Does this render the foods completely safe? It will take more than a decade of studies before we know for sure.

A healthier method for handling these types of meat products, called 'The Wisconsin Process,' uses lactic acid in place of the harmful nitrites and nitrates. The discovery was announced in mid-1986, but don't look for meats processed by this method any time soon. The industry says it is cost-prohibitive.

Further, although the ACS does not include alcoholic beverages on their list of nitrosamine-containing foods, it is important to note here that some whiskies and all beers also contain nitrosamines. If alcoholic spirits are high on your list of priorities, you might want to consider switching to the colorless varieties, such as gin and vodka, which do not have nitrosamines. To round out the list of offending goodies in this category, we must also add pickled foods. Do you really need that fatty corned-beef sandwich with a dill pickle on the side?

FLAME BROILING — The luscious smoke-flavored meat barbecued over hot charcoal or wood coals (or gas) that's an entrenched part of Americana also poses a danger. When the fat melts and drips onto the coals, producing the smoke that so deliciously flavors the meat, it also produces potential carcinogens.

The PAH chemicals in the smoke that coat the meat are a very real threat to health. These compounds are similar to the tars inhaled by cigarette smokers. Authorities estimate that the quantity of harmful compounds we consume by eating just one flame-broiled steak is the same as if we sat down and smoked 600 cigarettes one after the other.

This information is not new. As long ago as 1775, a British scientist by the name of Sir Percival Pott discovered that chimney sweeps constantly exposed to the carbons in soot developed cancer. In the late 1800s, skin cancer in German laborers was tied to their work with coal tars. Coal tar is still used to produce cancer experimentally in laboratory animals.

SMOKED FOODS — Smoked foods, including lox (smoked salmon), other fishes, ham, poultry and cheeses, absorb PAHs during the curing process. The level of harmful compounds is lower in these processed foods than is created by direct flame broiling, but many smoked foods are also preserved by the addition of sodium nitrate (see above).

In areas of the world where smoked foods are commonly found on the menu, there are documented higher incidences of cancer. In both the U.S.S.R. and Iceland, where the populations are undeniably fond of smoked fish, gastric cancer rates in particular are extremely high.

MUTAGENS — Mutagens are not just something you find in a science fiction movie. A mutagen is any agent which is able to cause a change in the basic structure of genes. Many medicines, chemicals, and physical agents (radiation, ultraviolet light) have the ability to induce a genetic mutation. However, what we are primarily concerned with in this chapter are the carcinogenic mutagens which have been found in wide variety in cooked, smoked, roasted, and browned foods.

Research conducted by Dr. Barry Commoner at the Center for the Biology of Natural Substances, Washington University, revealed the presence of mutagens in coffee (roasted), hamburgers (as prepared in most fast-food facilities), and in many commercially processed foods. Commoner's research showed that meat developed mutagens when cooked at temperatures over 300 degrees F., as well as when the meat was in contact with metal for a long period.

Dr. Takashi Sugimura, a Japanese biologist, has determined that mutagens develop when the protein in food is heated. Dr. Sugimura has classified over a dozen mutagens produced when the proteins or amino acids are heated in the normal cooking process. Foods which produce mutagens in cooking include dairy products, cereals, potatoes, meat, fish and baked goods. Toasted bread (yes, our breakfast toast), french fried potatoes, black butter (named *beurre noire* in gourmet French cookery), and carmelized sugar all develop mutagens in the browning process. Science has yet to classify this type of mutagen as carcinogenic, but any substance able to do genetic damage is suspect. The experts say that the burned fat on roasted meat is another instance where the meat itself is bathed with potentially harmful chemicals as the fat melts and coats the meat during the roasting process. In addition, any overheated cooking oil which begins to smoke has developed harmful mutagens and should never be used to cook food.

PROTECT YOURSELF — If you insist on broiling meat, forego that flame-kissed flavor. The experts say that when the heat source comes from above the meat and not below it, the risk of ingesting the harmful chemical compounds is minimized. When the heat radiates down on the meat, the browning fat drips into the broiler pan. The fat thus does not sizzle and flame and the smoke which carries the carcinogenic hydrocarbons (PAHs) does not occur.

Washington University has determined that broiling meat under an electric element or using a microwave (without a browning plate) will reduce health risks dramatically. Meats cooked in this manner did not develop mutagens.

More good news is the fact that experimental studies show that when green vegetables are eaten at the same meal as fried/flame-broiled meat, a significantly reduced number of mutagens are excreted in the urine, indicating that the mutagens in the meat are neutralized to some degree by ingesting vegetables at the same time. After a meal of fried meat alone, mutagenic levels in the body are increased. This fact has been confirmed by urinalysis. This study clearly indicates that certain foods can protect against potentially carcinogenic heat-induced mutagens.

Therefore, science makes a strong case for serving and eating greens with any basic meat dish. Essential fatty acids (linoleic and linolenic), present in abundance in *unrefined* virgin linseed, pumpkin, soy, and walnut oils, plus certain antioxidants (Vitamins C and E, selenium), not only protect against mutagens, but against cancer as well. Along with the important vitamins, strong antimutagenic substances have been identified in wheat sprouts, leaf lettuce, brussel sprouts, mustard greens, cabbage, broccoli, and spinach. Popeye knew it all the time.

ADDITIONAL RISKS

TOBACCO — Smoking and/or chewing tobacco in any form is documented to be the biggest cancer risk factor of all. Tobacco contributes to 30 percent of *all* cancers and is the major cause of lung cancer. Those who chew tobacco are inviting both mouth and throat cancer. In addition, there is a mountain of research about the dangers of 'secondary smoke,' the smoke exhaled in a closed environment by smokers. Those who are forced to involuntarily inhale secondary smoke have a higher incidence of respiratory and allergic problems than a general mix of the population who don't live or work with smokers. (Please see Chapter 14 for more on tobacco.)

ALCOHOL — Alcohol transports carcinogens to the body's tissues and may foster tumor growth. In addition to the fact that certain alcoholic beverages contain nitrosamines, detailed earlier in this chapter, consuming alcohol regularly increases the risk of developing liver cancer. Studies show that even social drinkers who take more than two drinks daily on a regular basis are increasing their risk. Really heavy drinkers commonly develop first cirrhosis of the liver and then cancer. Even worse, drinking and smoking adds to the risk of contracting mouth, throat, larynx and esophagus cancer.

CONTAMINATES — If you are in the habit of cutting away a spot of mold from cheese or vegetables and then serving the rest, you're adding to your health risk. Molds are living organisms and have fine roots, invisible to the eye, which penetrate deep into the food. Just because penicillin was developed from a mold doesn't mean all molds are good-for-you antibiotics. It's best to throw out moldy foods immediately.

SUNSHINE — Although the sun does help increase Vitamin D supplies in the body, too much sunshine not only ages the skin prematurely, but also causes skin cancer. If you work outside or insist on 'working on your tan' all summer, take steps to protect yourself from this very common form of cancer. The American Cancer Society says a sunscreen (at least #15) is mandatory and recommends a hat and long sleeves during the period from 11:00 a.m. to 3:00 p.m. when the sun is most fierce. ACS has also issued a warning against tanning salons, sunlamps, and tanning pills.

TANNING SALONS — Tanning parlors are springing up all over the country and are being heavily patronized by those who want the bronzed Hawaiian-vacation look all year around. Busy men and women, particularly those who operate on a tight schedule, find an hour a week in a tanning booth is enough to maintain a healthy-*looking* tan. But just how healthy is it?

Tanning lamps provide ten times the intensity of the noon sun in summer. They produce two types of ultraviolet light. One type, Ultra- violet A (UV-A), is the form which causes the skin to age rapidly. The other, Ultraviolet B (UV-B), is used by researchers to produce skin cancer in laboratory animals.

Salon owners respond to these facts by claiming to use lamps which generate 95 percent UV-A and just 5 percent UV-B, thereby reducing your risk of developing skin cancer. However, the intensity of the UV-A rays is practically guaranteed to age your skin prematurely. Once the deep-down damage is done, the condition is permanent. There is no known 'cure' which will restore the ability of the skin to produce the elastin and collagen necessary to keep it healthy, supple, and young.

In addition, UV-A light can react adversely with certain medications and may cause a severe allergic reaction. If you are on antibiotics, antihistamines or antidepressants, check with your doctor before scheduling a tanning session. An outbreak of itchy red welts all over your body is uncomfortable and unsightly, no matter how beautifully bronzed you are.

Another drawback of a tanning booth tan is the need to wear the protective goggles provided by the salon. UV-A rays can burn the cornea of the eye and cause irreversible damage. And that unavoidable white ring around the eyes is a dead giveaway that your tan came from a salon and not the French Riviera. The 'racoon look' will never be fashionable.

MICROWAVES — As documented earlier in this chapter, microwave cooking of meat is far safer than flame-broiling. But in light of other evidence regarding electromagnetic radiation, this may be a case of ,darned if we do and darned if we don't.'

Although American scientists still refuse to commit on whether microwaves and other electromagnetic radiation sources increase our cancer risks, laboratory rats exposed to levels equating to the maximum levels currently considered acceptable in the U.S. for humans did develop tumors. Researchers at the Bioelectromagnetics Research Laboratory of the University of Washington tested the 100 rats so exposed, looking for malignancies as well as changes in behavior, blood chemistry, and metabolism. At the close of the 25 month study, they discovered 16 tumors in the exposed rats, but only 4 in the control group. Most of the cancerous tumors were in the endocrine system.

The Environmental Protection Agency has blocked regulation which would have limited the strength of radio and television transmitters, currently monitored on a voluntary basis by the industry, on the grounds that further testing is needed to determine safe levels of electromagnetic radiation on humans.

The agency apparently does not believe that levels of exposure on average pose a risk great enough to allow regulation at this time.

However, a Virginia Commonwealth University microwave expert, Stephen Cleary, points out, "Nobody really knows what the safe levels are." Cleary cautions that more and more sources of electromagnetic radiation, such as the new cellular telephones, are entering the market place. (see *Electrical Fields* and *Geopathogenic Zones* Chapter 11.)

WATCH OUT FOR — Excessive x-rays, long-term use of hormones, and exposure to certain harmful chemicals and fibers (such as photocopy and photographic chemicals, asbestos). They are all potential additional risks. Question your physician about the need for x-rays; there may be another diagnostic tool he can use instead. Don't take hormones any longer than necessary. If your work involves you with carcinogenic chemicals and/or fibers, wear protective clothing, follow safe procedures, and learn emergency measures.

THE CLINCHER

If you're still skeptical of the importance of following good dietary practices, the results of a massive Chinese study on the relationship diet plays in preventing cancer should convince you.

Dr. T. Colin Campbell, Professor of Nutritional Biochemistry at Cornell University, and Dr. Jun-shui Chen of Beijing (Peking), China acted as co-directors of the project. This incredible undertaking actually began in the mid-1970s when 96.7 percent of the mainland China population, upwards of 800 million people, were surveyed by 650,000 Chinese workers to determine the death rate from cancer.

Dr. Campbell entered the picture in 1980 when he learned of the extraordinary data the Chinese had accumulated from Dr. Chen, then doing postgraduate work at Cornell. In 1983, Dr. Campbell and Dr. Chen designed and implemented the current diet/cancer study. Using the invaluable material from 1975 as a starting point, researchers were able to test 13,000

Chinese in rural areas of the country, all of whom ate local foods and lived in communes.

The resulting data from the 10-year study has provided powerful and conclusive evidence of the important part nutrition plays in preventing cancer. We invite you to consider the following facts and make your own determination.

Fact: In communes where more meat protein was eaten, the Chinese had significantly higher incidences of colorectal cancer, cancer of the lung, and more often fell victim to leukemia than those who ate less of the suspect forms of protein. Those who ate higher levels of protein also had a higher death rate from cancers of the esophagus and stomach.

Fact: The Chinese who had a higher intake of Vitamin A were protected against cancer of the esophagus and stomach.

Fact: Communes with a higher intake of Vitamin C suffered less incidence of terminal esophageal and stomach cancers.

Fact: Higher beta carotene levels resulted in a lower death rate from cancer of the stomach and esophagus.

Fact: The study showed that villages where selenium intake was up had a lower rate of cancer of the stomach and esophagus.

Fact: The communal village where serum cholesterol levels were tabulated highest had a whopping 473 times as many dying from cancer of the esophagus as the villages with the lowest cholesterol levels. High cholesterol levels also accounted for more deaths from leukemia, lung, colon, rectal, and stomach cancers than communes where cholesterol levels were lower. (See *Cholesterol* this chapter).

Fact: Villages where the diet was higher in fiber (up to 57 grams per day) had an overall lower death rate from all types of cancer than communes where fiber consumption was low (as little as 3 grams per day).

Presenting their findings before the American Society for Clinical Nutrition at the annual 1985 meeting, Dr. Campbell stressed that the work of correlating all the data has only just begun. Most likely the final analysis and report will be released for publication sometime this year.

However, it is very clear that even these few preliminary facts provide conclusive evidence of the importance of planning a dietary program which incorporates the documented cancer-preventive factors available to us all. Here's a quick review of the important points presented in this chapter.

GENERAL DIETARY GUIDELINES SHOWN TO LOWER YOUR RISK OF DEVELOPING CANCER (& HEART PROBLEMS)

1. Eat a variety of vegetables, fruits, berries, and nuts.

2. Insure an adequate intake of vitamins and minerals by choosing whole foods instead of refined, overprocessed foods.

3. Plan menus around whole grains, vegetables, and fruits that are high in complex carbohydrates and fiber to promote healthy bowel function.

4. Decrease your intake of saturated animal fats and chemically-altered fats (margarine, processed vegetable oils, salad dressings, shortening).

5. Eat three servings of fish each week. Choose poultry and low-fat dairy products often. Reduce your consumption of fatty red meat.

6. Learn to enjoy a leafy green salad with plenty of raw vegetables. Cooked foods should be baked or steamed, instead of fried or grilled.

7. Cut down on salt by using lemon, herbs, and spices instead.

8. Eat a lot of fresh whole foods, or choose those which have been only minimally processed.

9. Avoid cured, pickled, and traditionally smoked foods.

10. Avoid eating moldy foods. (This includes cutting off moldy edges.)

11. If you enjoy alcoholic drinks, keep your consumption moderate.

12. Maintain an appropriate body-weight. Avoid high calorie foods devoid of nutrients. Learn to love whole-grain cereal products, fruits, and vegetables.

Chapter V

The Importance of Dietary Fats

The Essential Fatty Acids vs The Destructive Fats

Both the National Cancer Society and the American Heart Association have stated that, in general, the average daily fat consumption of the American people is excessive. These two organizations, both dedicated to improving the health of the nation, have issued dietary guidelines which strongly suggest that we can reduce our risk of developing cancer (and the other degenerative diseases) simply by trimming (at least) 10 percent of the fat from our daily menus and eating lean.

On the surface of it, this seems to be an easy guideline to observe. It's really not difficult for the family cook to skim off the fat that rises to the top of the pot when making soups, stews, and gravies. A fish sauced with lemon and herbs is even more delicious than a greasy hamburger, and a lot healthier. Every supermarket in the country carries well-known and heavily advertised name brands of margarines and vegetable oils that proudly claim to be free of the saturated fats that promote harmful blood cholesterol levels. Every refrigerator case in every supermarket in every locale holds a vast selection of low-fat dairy products. Even salad dressings and mayonnaises especially processed to be low in fat are now readily available.

But — *and it's a big but* — just how healthy are these commercially processed fats and oils? Because medical researchers and scientists all over the world have found that the excessive consumption of dietary fats can be dangerous to our health, we decided to do some serious in-depth digging to find out the *real* story behind the brief dietary guidelines suggesting a reduction in fats which have been issued in recent years.

FATS & OILS IN HISTORY

Mankind has used the natural fats for both food and other purposes since prehistoric times. There is evidence showing that the early Egyptians made use of olive oil in flavoring, preparing, and preserving foodstuffs, as well as using it as a lubricant in moving the immense building blocks of the ancient pyramids. They also made a very efficient axle grease from fat and lime. As far back as 1400 BC, Homer tells us that oil was an aid to the weaver. Pliny mentions both hard and soft soaps, made with wood ashes and fats. In Biblical times, olive oil was so highly regarded that it was used in preparing offerings to the Lord (Leviticus 2:1), and for holy annointings (Exodus 30:22), as well as gracing the family table as a worthy staple of life.

THE OIL PROCESSING INDUSTRY — The industry as we know it has been growing by leaps and bounds for over fifty years. However, medical detectives and scientists have made some startling discoveries in the past two decades about the way fat metabolism works (or doesn't work) in the body. Perhaps if we had known fifty years ago what we know *now* about the ways in which chemically altered fats lead irrevocably to a host of degenerative diseases, the government might have taken a different position on these products. According to reliable sources, the methods used by the commercial oil industry to manufacture dietary fats are subject to 'periodic' review and re-evaluation by the Food & Drug Administration. In light of the growing masses of clinical research about the harmful effects of excessive fat intake, perhaps it's time to call for the FDA to exercise their prerogatives and do a thorough review of industry manufacturing methods in order to update their records.

In the so-called civilized societies, the increased incidence of the degenerative diseases (cancer, cardiovascular disease, diabetes, multiple sclerosis, liver and kidney problems) have paralleled the increased consumption of unnatural chemically altered fats. That may be a bold statement, but it's easily documented. A whopping 57 percent of our dietary fat consumption now comes from commercially processed fats and oils, such as margarine, shortening, salad, and cooking oils. At the turn of the century, cancer claimed the life of one person in every thirty, but today it kills one in five. One hundred years ago, heart disease took one person in every seven. The cardiovascular toll is now one person in every two.

DESTRUCTIVE 'INDUSTRIAL STRENGTH' FATS

You may find it hard to believe what the commercial oil industry does with some perfectly natural seeds before you find the finished products (margarine, cooking and salad oils, shortening) on the shelves of your neighborhood grocery stores. Here's what happens:

'COLD-PRESSED' — After the seeds are cleaned, they are mechanically crushed and subjected to fierce temperatures (the average is around 248 degrees F.) in order to break down the cell walls, thereby making the extraction of the oil easier. Because the vital live enzymes cannot survive temperatures much over 110 degrees F., it's already too late to save the enzymes, but we're just beginning. Next, the unappetizing dead mash of cooked seeds is forced through a giant press that works very much like an old-fashioned kitchen meat grinder. The difference is that this press exerts tremendous pressure (up to several tons per square inch). As the screw inexorably turns, the seeds are crushed and forced against the press head. This friction generates more heat (up to 203 degrees F.). This combination of friction-generated heat and press-crushing forces the seed to give up its oil.

If the processing stops here, these oils are allowed to be sold (usually in health-food stores at a premium price) as 'cold-pressed,' 'natural,' 'crude,' or 'unrefined.' Most authorities agree that the temperatures generated in the processing are high enough to cause deterioration of the essential fatty acids. As hard as it may be to believe, these 'cold-pressed' oils are the highest quality currently available from U.S. manufacturers.

'UNREFINED OIL' — Another favored method of extraction consists of using a chemical solvent to leach the oil from seeds. After being crushed and cooked, the seeds are then mechanically ground and processed with a chemical solvent at temperatures of up to 149 degrees F. (One popular solvent is *hexane,* manufactured from petroleum). You should know that the solvent is reclaimed after batches of seeds have been processed and is reused many times. Oils extracted with chemicals are unavoidably tainted with traces of these chemicals. Very often, chemically extracted oils are mixed with 'cold-pressed' oils. These oils find their way to stores and are marketed as 'unrefined oils.'

YOU ASKED FOR IT

Consumers have been brain-washed into believing that their salad and cooking oils should be clear, free-pouring at any temperature, odorless, and tasteless. Without commercial processing, natural oils offer the delicate taste characteristic of the seeds from which they came. They range in color from a pale yellow to gold to amber to almost red. Their different aromas are as distinctive as their different tastes. If you put them in the refrigerator, they become cloudy and their viscosity changes. In other words, they become somewhat heavier and thicker.

THE REFINING PROCESS — The first step in refining the oil, called degumming, is to remove most of the remaining phosphatides, essential for life. Lecithin (an important unsaturated fatty acid) is taken out. All the complex carbohydrates, some elements similar to proteins, and the gums are removed. The chlorophyll, calcium, magnesium, iron, and copper (health-promoting minerals) are also refined out.

Second, some caustic corrosive chemicals, such as sodium hydroxide (better known as Draino), or a mixture of sodium hydroxide and sodium carbonate, are dumped into the oil. The nasty mess is then mechanically agitated at a temperature of approximately 167 degrees F. The remaining free fatty acids combine with the caustic chemicals to form easily removed 'soaps.' Just about all that's left of the remaining minerals, protein-like elements, and phospholipids (fats with phosphorous and nitrogen), are eliminated during this stage of the 'refining' process. But the oil may be yellowish or reddish in color, still hanging on to a little of its identity in the form of pigments.

The third step consists of bleaching out the natural pigments to provide you with that colorless oil you've been taught to expect. Beta-carotene (a documented cancer-preventive) and chlorophyll, along with the last traces of the fatty acids, are filtered out, usually with acid-based clays, at temperatures of up to 230 degrees F. The essential fatty acids still present are further chemically damaged and may form toxic peroxides.

Deodorizing is the fourth step in the refining process. You couldn't possibly recognize the seed source of the oil at this point. The delicate flavor and scent that Mother Nature puts into her seeds has been replaced by unappetizing chemical odors and tastes. Taking out the bad taste and smell is accomplished by the use of a steam distilling process at extremely high temperatures (up to 518 degrees F.) for a period lasting as long as an hour. Thankfully, the dangerous peroxides and toxins produced in the previous step are removed, along with some of the pesticide residue. But the deodorizing process also eliminates the Vitamin E. *And,* of immense concern to all of us, the essential fatty acids have been transformed into something completely foreign to the human body.

The tortured oil must undergo yet another couple of steps before you buy it and take it home. Because the natural antioxidants (beta-carotene and Vitamin E) have been removed from the oil in the 'refining process,' synthetic chemical antioxidants are pumped in to lengthen the shelf life and a 'defoamer' is also added. And, because some of us refrigerate our salad and cooking oils, it is usually subjected to a process known in the industry as 'winterization.' The oil is artifically cooled and filtered yet again to insure that it remains clear under refrigeration. (This is the 'polyunsaturated oil' that is commonly added to commercial baby-formulas to provide 'essential fatty acids.')

The end result is an oil that is clear, odorless, tasteless, and indistinguishable from any other oil manufactured in the same manner. Unless the label tells you, there's absolutely no way to tell what the original seed source might have been. With all the vitamins and minerals eliminated, and the essential fatty acid molecules chemically altered, that oil on your supermarket shelves is a highly questionable food item.

ADDING INSULT TO INJURY

THE HYDROGENATION PROCESS — Even if the industry started with a completely natural oil (and they don't, they start with a chemically altered oil), the hydrogenation process destroys all nutritional value. Hydrogenating the oil consists of completely saturating all of the fatty acids with hydrogen. Hydrogenation is accomplished under pressure by using temperatures of up to 410 degrees F. in the company of a metal catalyst (nickel, platinum, copper) for as long as eight hours. Because the final product is a completely inert (dead) substance, it doesn't spoil and can be heated for (or in) cooking without becoming dangerously toxic. But it contains chemically altered bits of fatty acids, some of which may be harmful, and traces of the metal catalyst.

PARTIAL HYDROGENATION — By controlling the length of the hydrogenation process, a liquid oil can be transformed into a solid or semi-solid mass of fat. When the desired degree of hardness is attained, the hydrogenation process is stopped. Margarines and solid shortenings are manufactured with partially hydrogenated oils. Although logically you might not think so, *partially* hydrogenated products are actually more dangerous to your health than *fully* hydrogenated products. Here's why:

The molecules in the oil being bombarded with hydrogen become saturated (hydrogenated) erratically, leaving behind a proliferation of strangely altered substances when the process is halted. Many of these chemically alien elements are identified as being harmful because they interfere with the body's normal metabolism. Many others have not been scientifically researched and we just don't know what dangers they may pose when ingested.

MARGARINE — The Encyclopedia Britannica tells us that French chemist Hippolyte Mege-Mouries invented 'artificial butter' back in 1869. Mege-Mouries won the prize offered by Napoleon, who wanted a cheap fat to feed his soldiers and sailors, with his combination of skim milk and suet (melted beef fat). Although this disagreeable early butter substitute tasted just as awful as it sounds, it caught on. Mege-Mouries secured a patent for his process in the United States in 1873 and the industry as we know it today began.

As time passed, the animal fats used in the beginning gave way to imported vegetable fats, usually cottonseed, soybean, peanut, and corn oils, and the product became more palatable. The early manufacture of margarine was subject to strong restrictive legislation in the U.S. because both the butter producers and the nation's farmers feared for their livelihood. However, during the 1930s, U.S. farmers began supplying cottonseed and soybeans and the fledgling 'artificial butter' industry was on its way. As recently as the World War II years, margarine was sold uncolored. The white block, looking like a brick of shortening, came with a packet of powdered yellow-orange dye which the housewife had to blend in, usually by squeezing it through the softened mass with her hands.

No matter what seed oil the margarine manufacturer starts with, and usually the cheapest source is used, the essential fatty acids present to start with are either destroyed or changed in the hydrogenation process into chemically altered substances. The essential fatty acids that remain fight with the carbon fatty acids and reduce the nutritional value of the essentials still further. Add to this the fact that the minerals and vitamins the body needs for efficient metabolism of fats were ,refined' out and you have a nearly indigestible fat.

A very efficient advertising campaign has led us to believe that margarine is good for us because it's made with polyunsaturated fats. We equate polyunsaturates with good health because we know that the essential fatty acids are polyunsaturates. But what they don't tell us is that the polyunsaturates in margarine are *not* the essential fatty acids the body cries out for, but chemically altered alien fats. It is true that margarine contains no cholesterol, but the presence of so many chemicals completely alien to the body cancels out that small advantage. Remember, there is a lot of evidence showing that these chemically altered fats are strongly implicated in the degenerative diseases.

HOW MUCH IS TOO MUCH? — A lot of very authoritative medical scientists hold the position that the body reacts adversely to even a smidgin of a chemically altered alien substance. The cumulative effects of regularly consuming a diet high in chemically altered fats are devastating.

Studies show that hard margarines contain an average of over 30 percent chemically altered fatty acids. (Some brands register a whopping 60 percent.) Soft margarines (and diet margarines) contain an average of close to 20 percent chemically altered fatty acids. The measureable *essential* fatty acids present in margarines are virtually zero — less than 5 percent in all brands tested.

Hard vegetable shortenings tallied an average of 20 percent chemically altered fatty acids, with some brands containing close to 40 percent. Vegetable salad oils contain nearly 15 percent chemically altered fatty acids.

Commercially made baked goods average nearly 35 percent chemically altered fatty acids. Candies contain close to 40 percent chemically altered fatty acids. Even that old standby, peanut butter, contains varying amounts of chemically altered fatty acids. I hate to tell you about french fries (up to 40 percent) and potato chips (another 40 percent).

IS BUTTER BETTER? — Cattle, goats, and sheep have been kept by man for the production of milk and milk products for as long as history has been recorded, and probably even earlier than that. As far back as 1200 BC, Hindu writings mention the use of butter as food. The early Europeans used butter, not as a food, but as a remedy for skin injuries and sore eyes. It was also widely used as a hair oil and as fuel for lamps.

Is butter better than margarine? Well, it is certainly natural and certainly *tastes* better. Unfortunately, of the 500 fatty acids which have been identified in butter, only a very small percentage are the essentials (linoleic acid 2%, linolenic acid, trace). Over 65 percent of butter's fatty acid content requires the same elements for metabolism as the essentials. If the non-essential fatty acids outnumber the essentials, it's easy to understand that the non-essentials will win the metabolic battle. Butter also contains a small (less than 5 percent) amount of chemically altered fatty acids. Unlike the chemically processed fats and oil discussed earlier, these altered fats are produced in the cow itself and are not a serious health risk.

Butter does contain about 1 gram of cholesterol in every pound. We're going to tell you the truth about cholesterol, required by every cell in the body, a little later in this chapter. For now, what you should remember is that the average diet is sadly lacking in the elements (essential fatty acids, certain vitamins and minerals) needed to process cholesterol efficiently. The natural diet consumed by our ancestors had these elements in abundance.

Another drawback is that our modern-day butter also registers the presence of unwanted pesticides and antibiotics. The cows feed on grasses and grains that are pesticide-treated. Antibiotics are routinely given to the animals themselves and commercially manufactured feed is treated with antibiotics. The target is harmful disease-promoting bacteria, which are destroyed by the antibiotic treatment. But some friendly bacteria have developed resistance to the drugs. With good reason, researchers fear that the resistance factor can cross over to the dangerous bacteria, making them less susceptible to antibiotics.

In favor of butter, we must point out that it can be used in and for all types of cooking without breaking down into dangerous toxins. It is stable in the presence of light, heat, and oxygen. The relatively small percentage of naturally-occurring altered fatty acids is not a threat to health, but you can't depend on butter for your supply of essential fatty acids. Butter is easy to digest and the cholesterol content is not harmful, as long as your diet contains the elements necessary for the efficient metabolism of fat. However, even this natural dietary fat can create problems when consumed in excess. To sum it all up, butter *is* better for you, unless you're a glutton about it.

It's important to remember that fatty acids are essential to life. They play a vital part in the functioning of the entire body. It's therefore very important to seek out and incorporate good sources of the right kind of fatty acids into your daily diet. The following diagram illustrates the relationships of polyunsaturated dietary fatty acids and their influence on human diseases.

Presence of Polyunsaturated Fatty Acids in Various Oils and Their Influence on Human Diseases.

OILS

Flax (Linseed)	— A
Safflower	— B
Sunflower	— C
Corn	— D
Olive	— E

OMEGA-3 FATTY ACID (Linolenic)

A — Flax (Linseed)	—	58%
B — Safflower	—	0%
C — Sunflower	—	0%
D — Corn	—	0%
E — Olive	—	0%

THE FORMATION OF

Prostaglandins and Leukotrienes

PREVENTION OF

Flax oil (linseed oil) is the oil with the highest known content of Omega-3 fatty acids of all vegetable oils.

Omega-6 and Omega-3 families of dietary long chain unsaturated fatty acids are of clinical interest as has been explained in this chart.

This chart has been done in such a manner as to portray in laymen's terms the association of the essential fatty acids and their relation to human diseases.

Atherosclerosis and Arteriosclerosis
Arthritis
Cancer
Thrombosis
Asthma
Various Heart Diseases

OMEGA-6 FATTY ACID (Linoleic)

A — Flax (Linseed)	—	14%
B — Safflower	—	75%
C — Sunflower	—	65%
D — Corn	—	59%
E — Olive	—	8%

THE FORMATION OF

Prostaglandins and Leukotrienes

CONTRIBUTION TO

Flax oil (linseed oil) is the best seed oil for people with fatty degeneration, because the oil contains the largest amount of the most strongly dispersing essential fatty acid, the three times unsaturated linolenic acid (LNA = linolenic acid = Omega-3).

LNA helps to disperse from our tissues deposits of the saturated fatty acids and cholesterol, which like to aggregate and which make platelets sticky. (Platelets play an important role in blood coagulation and blood thrombus formation.) The oil has to be fresh, and not exposed to light, oxygen, and heat, because these three agents destroy the essential fatty acids very rapidly. Flax oil (linseed oil) should be *unrefined.*

*From "Fats and Oils — The Complete Guide to Fats and Oils in Health and Nutrition," by Udo Erasmus, Alive Books, Vancouver, B. C.

THE MYSTIQUE OF CHOLESTEROL — There are so many misconceptions and half-truths surrounding the workings of cholesterol in the human body that it seems like a good idea to remind you that cholesterol is required by every cell in the body *and* is the raw material from which the body produces bile acids, certain hormones, and provitamin D3. Simply eliminating cholesterol from the diet doesn't work. The body can manufacture up to about 1½ grams of cholesterol every day, and does, if it isn't supplied in the diet. It really isn't the level of cholesterol in the blood that creates health problems, it's whether the body has the elements it needs to process it properly.

THE IMPORTANT FATS

Because we're already on the subject of cholesterol, it seems appropriate to again explain the relationship between the essential fatty acids and cholesterol here. Cholesterol is dissolved and held in suspension in a free-flowing liquid state in the blood in the presence of adequate essential fatty acids. Because the melting point of cholesterol is 300 degrees F., it is deposited on arterial walls as an insoluble substance at the normal body temperature of 98.6 degrees F. With the fatty acid *lecithin* present, the melting point of cholesterol is reduced to 180 degrees F., still insoluble at body temperature. But when the essential fatty acids *linoleic* and *linolenic* are in sufficient supply, the melting point of cholesterol comes down to 32 degrees F., well below normal body temperature. In a liquid state, cholesterol cannot end up as harmful arterial plaque and does not promote the degenerative diseases.

FISH OIL — There's been a lot written lately about the omega-3 fatty acids (*eicosapentaenoic acid* (EPA) and *docosahexaenoic acid* (DHA) present in the arterial-cleansing fish oils. The fact that Eskimos and the Scandinavian peoples eat a lot of cold-water fish (rich sources of EPA and DHA) and enjoy a very low incidence of degenerative disease led researchers to study the workings of these two highly unsaturated fatty acids in the body. It was determined that EPA and DHA help lower the melting point of the saturated fats, thus keeping them from attaching themselves to arterial walls.

The important polyunsaturated fatty acids of marine origin enter the human food chain via a simple process. They are formed naturally in underwater plants and organisms, such as phytoplankton and algae. Many fish feed on these sea creatures and other larger fish, in turn, feed on them. As these elements are incorporated into the flesh of marine life, the fatty acids are welcomed into their lipid structure. The fish oils that are important to human life are present in their purest and most concentrated form in the fish that swim in the cold oceans of the world. Science says that it is the low temperature of this environment which dictates that their fatty acids should be of the highly unsaturated type.

However, the oils of many marine species contain toxic fatty acids which are harmful to humans. Cetoleic acid, shown to foster fatty degeneration of the heart, is present in herring oil, cod liver oil, and the oils of menhaden and anchovetta. And warm-water species and lean low-fat fish may be tasty and nutritious, but don't provide the important omega-3 fatty acids that protect against heart disease and cancer.

The world's leading authority on the omega-3 fatty acids present in marine oils is acknowledged to be the brilliant Danish professor, J. Dyerberg, M.D., Ph.D. Dr. Dyerberg heads the Department of Clinical Chemistry at the Aalborg Hospital (Aalborg, Denmark) and is responsible for a number of landmark papers on the effects of the polyunsaturated fatty acids, particularly in the treatment and prevention of atherosclerosis.

Dr. Dyerberg has an explanation for the failure of most nutritional authorities to recommend the daily intake of marine oils until recently. He says, "Fish oils were originally not mentioned in most dietary guidelines to lower serum cholesterol and prevent atherosclerosis. One reason for this might be that the populations most concerned with preventing atherosclerotic diseases do not readily accept and enjoy eating seafood. Another reason is that the long-chain polyunsaturated fats have low melting points and are easily oxidized. These qualities create problems in the manufacture of margarine and shortening. Reports published in the 1950s and 1960s indicating that fish oil may lower blood cholesterol even more than vegetable oil had no major impact on early dietary recommendations. The first real breakthrough concerning dietary fats occurred with the report of the clinical effects on coronary atherosclerosis of a diet rich in seafood."

In conjunction with H. O. Bang, it was Dr. Dyerberg who initiated the dietary studies of the Greenland Eskimos in the late 1970s. This report was published in 1981 in *Acta Scandanavia* Vol. 210: 245-248. Building on earlier research, the scientists uncovered the reason for the very low incidence of cardiovascular disease in Eskimo society. Although the population ate a very high fat diet (known to promote heart disease) of whale, seal, and walrus meat, they universally consumed a lot of cold-water fish as well.

After expanding his study to include Greenlanders, Dr. Dyerberg explains, "Statistics from Greenland show a low mortality rate from ischemic heart disease (atherosclerosis) with no sex difference. From 45 to 64 years of age, 25 out of 277 male deaths (9 percent) and 13 out of 178 female deaths (7 percent), or 38 out of 455 deaths (8.4 percent) in both sexes were recorded in a 5-year period within a population of approximately 50,000. In the community of 2000 inhabitants which we studied, which had a hospital with ECG facilities, 10 years of medical records did not include a single death from ischemic heart disease."

Within the last few decades, cardiovascular disease has risen steadily in Japan. As the Japanese people have embraced western dietary preferences in place of their traditionally high consumption of fish, the rate of death from cardiovascular disease has kept pace. As they have dropped fish from the menu and patronize McDonald's instead, the Japanese no longer enjoy their previous immunity from heart disease. Western disease patterns are now apparent in the population of Japan.

Most of us would not find a daily diet of fish palatable. It would be difficult indeed for the typical American to choke down the amount of fish that gives the Eskimos their seeming immunity to heart disease. However, a Dutch scientist by the name of D. Kromhout recognized the problems such a diet would pose to the western world and had a study already in progress to determine exactly what quantity of fish a person would have to eat to enjoy its protective effect. The results of Kromhout's study were published in the *New England Journal of Medicine* in 1985. Here's what he found:

In order to calculate the relationship between the measured intake of fish and coronary mortality, Kromhout selectively chose a group of 852 middle-aged men whose dietary habits could be determined for the 20-year period of the study. He assigned risk factors according to the amount of fish normally consumed. Men who disliked fish and never ate it at all were found to have a risk factor of 1.0. Those men eating from 1 to 14 grams of fish had a risk factor of 0.64; those consuming 15 to 29 grams had a risk factor of 0.56; and those eating 30 to 144 grams of fish every day had a risk factor of 0.36. After reviewing Kromhout's data, Dr. Dyerberg noted, "The interesting observation made by Kromhout is the inverse relationship between a relatively low level of fish intake and coronary heart disease. This finding makes nutritional advice based on the seafood hypothesis much easier to give and accept, compared to that based on data from Greenland and Japan which describe fish intakes that are unrealistically high for many people."

HEART HEALTH & MUCH MORE — Both EPA and DHA are present in the most important and active organs and tissues of the body, including the brain cells, the nervous system, and the sex glands. The omega-3 fatty acids play a very important part in regulating the chemical balance of the body and assist in normalizing the coagulation factor of the blood. In impressive double-blind clinical studies, fish oil has been shown to possess remarkable arterial-cleansing ability. It has reduced cholesterol and triglyceride levels, markedly lowered dangerously high blood pressure, eased the pain of rheumatoid arthritis, worked against migraines, and has even shown protective effects against cancer. The researchers are onto something big. Here's what they're saying now:

Both the American Heart Association and the American Cancer Society have published research showing that the American diet is both excessively high in the wrong kinds of fats and woefully deficient in the right kinds of fats. Health experts around the world have documented the health problems arising as a result of consuming too much fat. Physicians routinely monitor cholesterol and triglyceride levels to determine those at high risk of suffering a heart attack.

Heart Disease: Cardiologists and doctors all over the world are now prescribing fish oils as a proven therapeutic measure for those with dangerously high cholesterol and triglyceride readings. In clinical tests, omega-3 fish oils were shown to almost miraculously lower harmful blood fats, while increasing beneficial blood fats that protect against heart disease.

In the *New England Journal of Medicine,* Dr. Michael Davidson of St. Luke's Medical Center reported on a study of patients taking fish oil capsules which showed spectacular results. Overall cholesterol levels dropped 24% and triglyceride levels fell 48%. Dr. Davidson pointed out that simply taking fish oil capsules cut the risk of suffering a fatal heart attack by 50% for these patients.

Cancer: Germany's premiere biochemist, Dr. Johanna Budwig favors a nutritional approach to the treatment of cancer. As an important part of the diet, she feeds her cancer patients freshly caught rainbow trout, a good source of the omega-3 fatty acids. Dr. Budwig has demonstrated the incredible tumor-dissolving effects of EPA, DHA, linolenic and linoleic acids in her practice and is noted for her seemingly miraculous cures of terminal cancer patients, extensively detailed in the following chapter (Chapter 6).

Studies indicate that a high-fat diet can foster cancer. But recent studies coming from Dr. Michael Pariza of the University of Wisconsin are beginning to alter scientific thinking. Dr. Pariza showed that 75 percent of lab animals fed a high-fat/HIGH-CALORIE diet got cancer, but only a tiny 7 percent of the animals fed a high-fat/LOW-CALORIE diet developed tumors. It has long been known that obesity adds to the risk

93

of cancer. Cutting fat from the diet is an efficient way to lose pounds, but cutting calories may be more effective.

New research shows that the omega-3 fatty acids actually suppress some cancer-promoting substances. Rutgers University researcher Dr. Rashida A. Karmali says early indications are that omega-3 may protect against breast and prostate cancer. Dr. Karmali says, "Animals given fish oil had a significantly lower rate of cancers when exposed to cancer-causing agents or when they received transplanted tumors." Other scientists have reported similar findings against colon and lung cancers.

Dr. William E. Connor, Oregon Health Sciences University: "There is more and more evidence indicating that omega-3 fatty acids have a fundamental role in human health, both as a necessary nutrient and to prevent certain diseases occurring as a result of a chemical imbalance."

Arthritis: Until now, medical science held out no real hope of curing arthritis. The treatment of choice consists mainly of giving anti-inflammatory drugs, such as aspirin, to reduce pain and swelling. British researchers recently discovered that the herb Feverfew works better than aspirin, has no harmful side effects, and the pain relieving anti-inflammatory benefits of Feverfew actually last longer.

Because both Feverfew and fish oils are natural food substances with no known harmful side effects, some authorities believe that a combination of the two could spell real relief for arthritics.

Another useful, completely natural adjunct to the treatment of arthritis are the omega-3 fatty acids. Joel M. Kremer, M.D. of Albany Medical College explains that a group of eicosanoids called leukotrienes have been identified as a possible cause of the pain and inflamed joints of rheumatoid arthritis. When the omega-3 fatty acids in fish oil are supplemented in the diet, the chemical composition of the leukotrienes becomes almost magically less inflammatory.

In a recent 12-week long double-blind study of arthritis patients, Dr. Kremer found that patients given 1.8 grams of a concentrated fish oil supplement reported greatly reduced pain and swelling. Calling the results "very encouraging," Dr. Kremer noted that the control patients in the study who were given an inert substance instead of fish oil showed no improvement.

Psoriasis: Because leukotrienes are believed to be responsible for the inflammation and scaling of severe psoriasis, some scientists are calling fish oil a possible treatment for this disfiguring skin disease. As reported in the *Annals of Allergy,* early British and U.S. studies report that fish oil supplements brought welcome relief to some (but not all) psoriasis sufferers.

Reducing Rejection: More good news from the *Journal of Surgical Research* reveals that a diet high in the omega-3 fatty acids lowers the risk of rejection when surgical tissue grafts are necessary. After noting this effect in laboratory animals, the scientists theorized that fish oil supplements work by altering the clotting factor of blood platelets, thereby reducing the body's rejection response to a foreign graft.

Overall: Dr. William Lands, Chief of Biological Chemistry, University of Illinois states: "We now understand the disease process much better and see that there is a dietary linkage. The potential for major improvements in health, not necessarily from a therapeutic point of view, but from a preventive medicine point of view, are really tremendous."

FISH OIL SUPPLEMENTS FLOOD THE MARKET — Certain fresh and salt water fish from icy cold northern waters have been determined to be excellent sources of EPA and DHA. In order of their importance, they are salmon, sardines, mackerel, trout, and eel. The omega-3 content of fresh salmon has been measured as between 18.9 percent and 31.4 percent of its total fat content. Lean low-fat fish, including pike, carp, and haddock, also contain EPA and DHA, but in minute quantities. The best source of the omega-3 fatty acids is salmon, but salmon is very expensive. Most of us wouldn't find it practical or even particularly pleasant to eat salmon every day. The easy way to add the protective effects of these wonder-working fatty acids to your daily diet appears to be as simple as selecting a good dietary supplement.

As more and more reports of the wonders of the omega-3 fatty acids have been picked up from the medical journals and trumpeted from the housetops, more and more manufacturers have come out with fish oil supplements. Unless you have considerable knowledge, choosing the right fish oil dietary supplement can be risky. For instance, if the fish oil in your capsule has been obtained from salmon (or trout) raised on a fish farm, the quality of the oil is inferior. The elements essential to the production of the omega-3 fatty acids in the fish are put in commercial fish foods, but deteriorate rapidly. Fish raised in a shallow tank or pond, in contrast to those swimming free and feeding on fresh, live marine animals and the rich vegetation of the sea, just cannot be considered a good source of EPA and DHA.

Another important point to consider when selecting a fish oil dietary supplement has to be the method of manufacture. EPA and DHA (and linolenic acid) are destroyed by light, air, and heat. These super-sensitive fatty acids must be handled delicately. Capsules must be filled quickly under stringent manufacturing procedures which insure that light, air, and heat are excluded. And the capsule shell must be opaque and dense enough to protect the precious contents from deterioration.

After doing an in-depth investigation of the fish oil products currently available, we have found what we believe to be the best fish oil supplement available anywhere. We think it's important to bring this little-known fish oil supplement to your attention.

Salmon Oil (from Biowell Co.), is a concentrated source of the important omega-3 fatty acids derived ONLY from salmon caught in the crystal-clear and pristine unpolluted waters off the Norwegian coast. Unlike many of the newly popular fish oil supplements, *Salmon Oil* is just that — pure salmon oil — not a conglomeration of mixed fish oils. This very special product has 1000 mg of salmon oil, each contains 120 mg EPA and 80 mg of DHA in each pure capsule. No sugar, starch, artifical Flavors or colors, chemical preservatives, yeast or sodium are added. You get pure deodorized salmon oil rich in omega-3 — and nothing else.

ONE FINAL OBSERVATION — Citing the work of German biochemist H. J. Mest ("The Influence of Linseed Oil Diet on Fatty Acid Pattern in Phospholipids & Thromboxane Formation in Platelets in Man," published in *Klin Wochenschr* in 1983), P.V. Johnston, Ph.D., of the University of Illinois (Urbana, Illinois), points out that Mest demonstrated an increase in the EPA and DHA content of serum phospholipids after several weeks of linseed oil supplementation.

Dr. Johnston says, "After four weeks, EPA was elevated 150 percent and DHA by 70 percent over initial levels." What this means is to you and me is that a *healthy* body can manufacture both EPA and DHA from linoleic acid, so they are not on the very exclusive list of essential fatty acids either. The problem is that few of us are housed in a truly healthy body working at optimum efficiency, so our production of EPA and DHA is inhibited. Let's tag EPA and DHA as very important fatty acids. *Arachidonic acid* is another important fatty acid, but most scientists agree that the body can produce arachidonic from linoleic acid. Therefore, it is not one of the true essentials.

However, as in most things, there is an exception which proves the rule. Laboratory studies of rats (reported in *Nutrition Reviews,* September 1986) show that the brain accumulates DHA and arachidonic acid quickly between birth and 20 days of age. This store correlates with a period of intense brain cell division. Between 20 and 40 days after birth, the rats show a heavy concentration of the fatty acids associated with the production of *myelin,* a protective sheath which covers all nerve fibers.

In an important paper entitled, "Fatty Acids in the Brain & Retina: Evidence for Their Essentiality," researchers M. Neuringer, Ph.D. (Oregon Health Sciences University and Oregon Regional Primate Research Center) and W. E. Connor, M.D. (Professor of Medicine, chief of the Division of Endocrinology, Metabolism & Clinical Nutrition, Oregon Health Sciences University, Portland, Oregon) explain how this relates to humans. "In human development, DHA and arachidonic acid accumulate rapidly both before and after birth. During the last trimester of pregnancy, cerebral and cerebellar content of these fatty acids increases three to five times; similar percent increases occur again between birth and twelve weeks of age.

"In primate (monkey) and human fetuses, levels of DHA and arachidonic acid are higher in the fetal blood than in maternal blood, whereas the opposite is true for their precursors, linolenic and linoleic acids. Selective incorporation mechanisms appear to exist to supply the fetal brain with the relatively high levels of DHA needed for normal development. After birth, newborn infants may be limited in their capacity to synthesize DHA and arachidonic acid from linolenic and linoleic acids and may be dependent on direct dietary sources. Human breast milk contains sufficient amounts of DHA and arachidonic acid to provide sufficient amounts for the developing brain. However, most synthetic human infant formulas provide no DHA or arachidonate. Infants fed these formulas have far less DHA in their blood fats than infants receiving human milk, even when ample linolenic acid is provided."

This is yet another bit of evidence showing that the mother who is able and nurses her child gives him a head start. A pregnant woman is well advised to make sure that her diet includes an adequate supply of these fatty acids, both while she is carrying the child and after delivery as well if she is planning to breastfeed her infant.

In the same paper, Drs. Neuringer and Connor point out that there is a growing body of evidence showing that EPA and DHA (of the n-3 group) should be classified as essential fatty acids on a par with linolenic acid (also an n-3 fatty acid), long known to be one of the true essentials. The scientists say that the n-3 fatty acids are important to the structure and function of membranes, particularly in the retina and central nervous system. Fish, shellfish, and marine mammals are a rich source of the n-3 fatty acids, including DHA, meaning that the body is not required to synthesize it.

In the body, high concentrations of DHA are present in the retina of the eye, the cerebral cortex of the brain, the testes and sperm. In fact, DHA makes up one-third of the fatty acid content of the cerebral cortex, explaining why fish has long been known as a 'brain food.' Because the body manufactures DHA from the essential fatty acids, the experts note that these high levels are automatically maintained by the body as long as dietary levels of the essential fatty acids are adequate. Studies show that deficiency symptoms can be reversed by supplying linolenic acid.

VEGETARIAN SOURCES OF OMEGA-3 FATTY ACIDS — *The New England Journal of Medicine* (Vol. 315, No. 13, 1986) recently published comments from A. P. Simopoulos, M.D. and N. Salem, Jr., Ph.D. (National Institute on Alcohol Abuse & Alcoholism) showing that *purslane* (Portulaca oleracea), a common garden herb which is better known as pigweed, is a good source of the omega-3 fatty acids. The authors point out that purslane is a common item on the menu in many Mediterranean countries which enjoy a low incidence of cancer and heart disease. They suggest that purslane could be a good source of the omega-3 fatty acids for vegetarians.

In the same issue, Michael A. Weiner, Ph.D. (Port Washington, New York) points out what he considers to be a drawback in the ingestion of fish oils. Dr. Weiner notes that, while dietary fish oils are prescribed for their antithrombotic and hypolipidemic effects, they contain a measure of cholesterol along with their healthy content of omega-3 fatty acids. However, because of the cholesterol-dissolving effect of EPA and DHA, many authorities discount this objection. Fortunately, for any of us who share Dr. Weiner's viewpoint, there are good plant sources of the omega-3 fatty acids. Dr. Weiner suggests that the botanicals might be a wiser choice for insuring that the important fatty acids are incorporated into the diet.

Because they are so important to your life and good health, it just makes good sense to plan meals which include the food sources of the important fatty acids. Before you do the family shopping, you might want to consult the following chart:

FOOD SOURCES & CELL DISTRIBUTION
OF THE FATTY ACIDS

Fatty Acid	Food Sources	Cell Distribution
*Linolenic Acid** n-3	Crude Vegetable Oils Linseed, Soy, Walnut, Pumpkin	Component of all cells
*Linoleic Acid** n-6	Crude Vegetable Oils	Component of all cells
EPA (Eicosapentaenoic Acid) n-3	Fish & Shellfish (cold-water varieties)	Minor component of all cells
DHA (Docosahexaenoic Acid) n-3	Fish & Shellfish (cold-water varieties)	Major component of brain, retina (eye) testes, and sperm
Arachidonic Acid n-6	Liver, Brain, Meats	Component of most membranes
Oleic Acid n-9	Animal & Vegetable Fats	Component of many cells (white matter/myelin)
Docosapentaenoic Acid n-3	None	Low in normal cells (replaces DHA in EPA & linolenic deficiency)
Eicosatrienoic Acid n-9	None	Accumulates in total EPA deficiency syndrome

* Essential Fatty Acids

THE ESSENTIAL FATTY ACIDS

Both *linoleic acid* and *linolenic acid are essential to life.* This means that the body must have these fatty acids to survive, but cannot manufacture them from other elements in the diet. They must be supplied daily in the foods we eat. We have already pointed out one very important function of the essential fatty acids (linoleic and linolenic). They keep cholesterol in suspension, thereby preventing the buildup of the arterial plaque associated with cardiovascular disease and fatty degeneration.

Another important function of linoleic and linolenic acid is the transport of oxygen throughout the body. Every cell (blood, tissue, organ) requires oxygen for functioning. When the membranes surrounding and protecting each cell are pumped full of oxygen, harmful bacteria cannot enter. Bacteria and viruses don't grow in the presence of oxygen. The essentials are fashioned to absorb sunlight energy, immeasurably enhancing their ability to carry oxygen.

Because the essentials possess a slight negative electric charge, their molecules repel one another. It is this factor which moves toxins to the detoxifying systems of the body (intestinal tract, kidneys, liver, lungs, skin) where they can be eliminated. The electric charge they carry is also very important to the workings of the heart, nerves, and muscles. Acting like Mother Nature's 'pacemaker,' the essentials regulate the all-important beating of the heart.

Essential fatty acids control chromosomes during cell division and are necessary to the formation of new cell membranes after a cell has divided. Because we know that cancer cells are abnormal cells which grow and perpetuate themselves by division, it's easy to understand why the essential fatty acids are so important as both a preventive and treatment of any form of malignancy.

Overall cancer prevention requires a thorough knowledge of the metabolic pathways through which cancer spreads, the vascular supply of various parts of the body, the relationship of adjacent organs, as well as a clear understanding of both the normal and altered functions of the body.

DEFICIENCIES ARE SERIOUS — Many health authorities are beginning to realize that essential fatty acid deficiencies are widespread. It has been shown that the tissues and blood levels of the victims of the degenerative diseases are lacking in the essential fatty acids. In many cases, even if the important fatty acids are present, the elements the body needs to put them to work are missing. This is called a 'functional deficiency.'

When the diet is lacking in the essential fatty acids, serious health problems develop. The killers (cancer, heart disease, and more) are fostered by an excessive intake of saturated fats (and chemically altered fats). Without the presence of the essential fatty acids, the killer diseases are given a very favorable environment. They thrive and grow, but we sicken and eventually die.

Other deficiency symptoms include liver and kidney degeneration, arthritis, circulatory problems, mood changes, vision complaints, hair loss, abnormal weakness, skin diseases, a lack of coordination, tingling in the extremities, inhibited growth, dryness of the mucous membranes (and glands), sterility in males, and miscarriages in females.

The September 1986 issue of *Nutrition Reviews* offers a clinical review of several cases of essential fatty acid (EFA) deficiency as observed in patients unable to take food by mouth and who were given fat-free TPN (total parenteral nutrition). A patient with short-bowel syndrome who was given fat-free TPN for 82 days showed all the classic symptoms of lineoleate deficiency. The article states: "Many of these patients had scaly skin (scleroderma), thrombocytopenia (an abnormal decrease in the number of blood platelets), and poor wound healing, accompanied by low levels of linoleic and arachidonic acid, and a high concentration of eicosatrienoic acid, strongly suggestive of linoleate deficiency."

When a female patient on fat-free TPN developed scleroderma, she was given 500 ml of plasma lipoproteins (fatty acids accompanied with red cell membranes) for a period of seven days. Her lipid values normalized promptly. In addition the visual disturbances which characterize an EFA deficiency were reversed simply by giving a linolenate-rich infusion.

Animal studies (National Academy of Science 1986) of monkeys showed that an EFA dietary deficiency produced retinal depletion of the n-3 fatty acids causing changes in vision. Pregnant female monkeys given a diet rich in safflower oil throughout their pregnancy, and to their infants after birth, exhibited sight abnormalities. An additional finding arising from this study indicates that the monkeys fed safflower oil had a reduced capacity for learning as well.

This important paper concludes with the suggestion that obstetricians and pediatricians should be aware that a linolenic deficiency of the pregnant mother is associated with visual and learning defects in the infant, especially if the infant's diet does not include sufficient EFA after birth.

The American Journal of Clinical Nutrition (Volume 44: September 1986) carried an article by E. M. Berry, M.D. MRCP and J. Hirsch, M.D. entitled "Does Dietary Linolenic Acid Influence Blood Pressure?" In this paper, Drs. Berry and Hirsch report on the long-term effects of polyunsaturated fats in the diet of 400 male subjects ranging in age from 20 to 78 years. They note that a mere one percent increase in dietary linolenic acid was associated with a corresponding healthy decrease in blood pressure.

This important work concludes, "Linolenic acid comprised only one-eighth the amount of linoleic acid, the major polyunsaturate in adipose (fatty) tissue and hence in the diet, yet it had a disproportionate association with BP (blood pressure). This may be related to its role as a precursor for the production of prostaglandins and/or other vasoregulators. Dietary manipulation with n-3 fatty acids may be helpful in the treatment and prevention of hypertension. Results suggest that linolenic acid, which is contained in linseed (flaxseed) oil, legumes, nuts, and citrus fruits, rather than linoleic acid may be the principle dietary polyunsaturated fatty acid related to blood pressure."

HOW MUCH IS ENOUGH? — Authoritative recommendations vary widely. How active you are physically, how stressed you are mentally, whether your daily diet is nutritionally correct, plus other factors personal to each of us, must all enter into an expert calculation of just how much of the essential fatty acids we individually need to consume every day. Most studies do agree, however, that males require up to three times as much of the essentials as females because of the differences in hormone production.

As a general rule of thumb, 9 to 30 grams daily (approximately 3 to 10 percent of the day's calories) of the essential fatty acids (linoleic and linolenic) seems to be about right for a normal person. Those of us who consume a diet high in saturated and chemically altered fats (and that includes the vast majority of the population), require the higher amount in order to rid the body of dangerous arterial plaque and gradually rebuild the cell and tissue damage caused by fatty degeneration.

Studies conducted with laboratory animals in which almost 30 percent of the day's calories were supplied in the form of linoleic acid resulted in no adverse changes in the animals over the long term, just as long as sufficient elements required for the processing of linoleic acid were also supplied. For efficient functioning, the body needs 1 part Vitamin E for every 1,500 parts linoleic acid. At the high end of the suggested daily allowance of essential fats (30 grams), around 50 I.U. of Vitamin E should be included in the diet. Other elements for efficient processing of the essential fatty acids include Vitamins A (or beta-carotene), C, B3, B6, and zinc.

FOOD SOURCES OF THE ESSENTIALS — As we have already discovered, the chemically altered fats present in common supermarket items like margarine, solid shortening, salad and cooking oils (and a lot of other commercially manufactured food products) are unhealthy in the extreme. You just cannot expect to get the essential fatty acids the body requires in these commercial products.

Be comforted. Mother Nature comes to the rescue with her delicious and very neatly packaged seeds and nuts. Remember, plants have the enzymes needed to manufacture the essential fatty acids, but man does not. It's no accident that the holy writings of many civilizations direct us to the plant kingdom, as in Ezekiel 47:12 —*"...and the fruit thereof shall be for meat."*

The very best and richest source of *both* the essential fatty acids (linoleic and linolenic) is *linseed oil.* (You're going to learn some incredible things about this oil a little later.) With 58 percent linolenic and close to 20 percent linoleic acid, linseed oil wins hands down, but there are a few other good natural sources as well. Pumpkin seed oil, soybean oil, and walnut oil contain both essentials, but are not as richly endowed as linseed oil. It is important that you know that these four sources provide the only oils which contain both essential fatty acids.

Olive oil, long a favorite of gourmets, contains no linolenic acid at all, and only 8 percent of its total fat content (20 percent) is present as linoleic acid. Also, despite what the manufacturers would like you to believe, corn oil contains not one trace of essential linolenic fatty acid. And, if you've been reading about safflower and evening primrose oil lately, you should know that they also contain only one of the essentials (linoleic acid), but offer no linolenic acid.

I almost hate to bring it up, but cottonseed, rapeseed, (commonly used in the commercial manufacture of vegetable oils, margarines, and solid shortenings) and peanut oil often contain toxins and toxic fatty acids. In addition, peanuts are easily contaminated by a toxic fungus that feeds on the damp legumes. (Strictly speaking, peanuts are not really nuts at all, but a member of the legume (bean pod) family.

NUTRITIONALLY PERFECT LINSEEDS

A nutritional analysis of this near-miraculous food reveals that mankind could very nearly sustain life on a diet consisting wholly of linseeds, probably more familiar to you as flax seed. Get ready for some surprising facts.

AMINO ACIDS — Linseed offers all of the essential amino acids, the ones the body requires but cannot manufacture. Replenishing the building blocks of life (proteins) is a daily requirement. If just one essential amino acid is missing from the diet, the resulting protein deficiency can lead to serious disease.

VITAMINS — Linseed is a rich source of the important fat-soluble Vitamins A, D, and E, plus B1, B2, and C (water-soluble). This should not come as a surprise. These are the vitamins the body needs to efficiently process the essential fatty acids. Even science is beginning to recognize that nature seldom slips up.

MINERALS — Linseed contains all the major minerals (potassium, phosphorus, magnesium, calcium, sulphur, iron, zinc, sodium, chlorine), plus the important trace minerals (manganese, silicon, copper, fluorine, aluminum, nickel, cobalt, iodine, aolybdenum, chromium). If you recognize that selenium and vanadium are not listed, chalk it up to the fact that very likely the seeds were not tested for these only recently identified minerals.

FIBER — Linseed is considered an excellent source of fiber, required for healthy intestinal and colon functioning. Fiber assists in removing cholesterol, softens the stool, and relieves constipation. The experts point out that a diet high in fiber helps cleanse the toxins from the blood and liver and goes a long way toward improving the quality of life as we age.

MUCILAGE — The old-fashioned name for glue may have been mucilage, but that doesn't apply here. This gelatin-like substance reduces excess stomach acidity, soothes and lines the mucous membranes of the digestive and intestinal tracts (assuring a smooth trouble-free passage of stool), and helps move cholesterol along. Because it acts to regulate the glucose content of the blood, mucilage is believed useful to the diabetic as well.

LINSEED OIL IS NUTRITIONAL GOLD

Oil pressed from linseeds is incredibly rich in both essential fatty acids. It carries between 15 and 25 percent linoleic acid (twice unsaturated) and from 50 to 60 percent linolenic acid (three times unsaturated). As we have already examined, both are essential to the life processes and must be supplied in the diet. Linseed oil is also a very good source of beta-carotene (a precursor of Vitamin A), Vitamin E, and lecithin (plus other phosphatides), all required for the efficient digestion of fats and oils.

The experts say that linseed oil also metabolizes to prostaglandins. Prostaglandins play an important part in the heart function, regulate blood pressure, and assist in arterial functioning. In addition, linseed oil steps up the metabolic rate and assists in the vital oxygenation of every cell in the body. Proponents point out that it's this factor which is responsible for the steady increase of energy and the feelings of exhilaration and 'lightness' that regular users of linseed oil (with high-quality protein) experience.

THE ESSENTIAL FATS + PROTEIN

THE MAGIC COMBINATION — It really shouldn't take hundreds of years of scientific research to determine the optimum diet. All we really have to do is get back to the basics and eat the basic natural foods our bodies were designed to process as fuel. We have already discovered that linseeds contain the essential fatty acids, *plus* high-quality protein, *plus* the elements the body requires to process the essential fatty acids. Mother Nature does it right.

TRACKING THE EVIDENCE — Today's medical researchers owe a great deal to a number of early German biochemists and scientists. The discoveries these men made, outlined below, served as a shining beacon showing the way to today's scientific truths. In 1842, the brilliant chemistry professor Baron Justus von Liebig published work showing the relationship between the essential fatty acids and protein. In rapid succession came the studies of Eduard Pflueger (physiologist) in 1875, Ernst F. Hoppe-Seyler (physician and founder of the first published biochemical journal) in 1876, and the noted biochemist Lebedow in 1888. Working with laboratory animals, Lebedow proved that severely malnourished and starving animals died more quickly on a diet high in protein (without fats) or high in fats (without protein) than when given no food at all. But when the animals were given quality fats and protein together, they quickly recovered. The high quality fat that Lebedow selected was linseed oil.

In 1899, the brilliant scientist Rosenfeld took up the cause. Rosenfeld's experiments proved conclusively that consuming only animal fats led inescapably to fatty degeneration of the inner organs and obesity. Because the research identifying the difference between saturated animal fats and the essential fatty acids was many years in the future, Rosenfeld didn't know *why* this was so, but he proved conclusively that it *was* so. As Rosenfeld continued with his work on nutrition, he discovered

107

in 1902 that consuming a diet high in carbohydrates and low in protein resulted in fat deposits, as does a high carbohydrate, high protein diet. However, when he added high quality fats to the menu, his subjects slimmed down, lost their fat deposits, and had increased energy into the bargain. Rosenfeld had confirmed Lebedow's theory of 'good' fats (linseed oil) versus 'bad' fats (animal fats).

In 1920, Otto Meyerhof (1922 winner of the Nobel Prize for Physiology & Medicine) discovered that linoleic acid and sulphur-rich proteins form a natural partnership in the body. It was his work on cellular oxygenation and the transformation of lactic acid in muscles, created by the combination of essential fats and quality protein, that won him international recognition, the Nobel Prize, and assured his place in the annals of medicine. Albert Szent-Gyorgyi, a naturalized American of Hungarian descent (standing alone in the midst of the advanced German scientists), took the Nobel in 1937 for his further research on biological oxidation and ascorbic acid (Vitamin C). His work confirmed that linoleic acid, when combined with sulphur-based proteins, stimulates the oxygenation processes of the body. The 1931 Nobel Prize in Physiology & Medicine went to Otto Heinrich Warburg for his research proving that quality fats were required to repair the oxygenation function when it was depressed by fatty degeneration resulting in cancer and/or diabetes.

It was not until the late 20s and early 30s that the essential fatty acids, as we know them today, were isolated and identified by the noted scientists G. O. Burr and M. M. Burr. The results of their important work were published in 1929 in the *Journal of Biological Chemistry* (Volume 82: 345-367) and updated in the *Journal of Biological Chemistry* in 1930 (Volume 86: 587-621). Here's what they discovered. Working with laboratory animals, these two biochemists proved that animals fed a high protein diet which is severely deficient in the essential fatty acids die quickly. If the condition is not too advanced, they also showed that recovery was swift when the essential fats were put back into the diet.

This very promising line of research was neglected as the age of specialization dawned. Instead of continuing on with combinations of nutrients as their predecessors had done, the scientists of 50 years ago (and for most of the intervening years) narrowed their field of endeavor and concentrated on one nutrient at a time. Amino acids received the bulk of their attention.

In the mid 1950s, another brilliant German scientist took up where all the others had left off. Dr. Johanna Budwig (you'll learn all about her astounding breakthroughs in the treatment of cancer and the other diseases of fatty degeneration in the following chapter) has been battling commercial interests for thirty years. Using a combination of linseed oil and sulphur-based proteins, Dr. Budwig has proven conclusively that a return to the natural ways of eating can cure cancer. Do you think that this information was eagerly accepted by a waiting world desperately searching for a cancer cure? Not on your life! Recognizing the dangers of commercially manufactured dietary fats (margarine, hard shortening, vegetable oils), Dr. Budwig sought to publicize her findings, but found her way blocked by German manufacturers with a heavy financial stake in these products.

Dr. Budwig retired from public life and opened her own practice. She depends entirely on nutritional correction for her documented successes in curing cancer cases given up as terminal by the oxthodox medical community. You will read all about her findings in the following pages.

Chapter VI
The Miracle of Linseed Oil

The Medicinal Fat

A very good friend, George Friedrich, suffered three serious heart attacks between the ages of sixty and sixty-three. At the rate of one heart attack every year, his doctors didn't hold out much hope for a complete recovery. George's entire cardio-vascular system was clogged with atherosclerotic plaque, interrupting the vital blood flow to his heart. He was put on very strong medication, including nitroglycerin for his angina pain, and was taking up to fifteen pills every day.

During the three years of his early sixties, George became very weak and aged visibly. He was on a downhill course until he was introduced to *Dr. Johanna Budwig's Formula*. He immediately incorporated Dr. Budwig's Formula into his daily diet. For breakfast every morning, he took 1 tablespoon of cold-processed, unrefined linseed oil mixed with low-fat cottage cheese. In order to make this fare more palatable, he added different herbs, raw vegetables, or fruits for variety. George found his favorite additions were a mixture of finely grated cucumbers and radishes with some chopped tomatoes.

After eating this low-fat cottage cheese 'salad' daily for just three months, George found his breathing was easing and the angina pain that had been with him for so long was almost eliminated. A year later, the medical doctors who examined him were amazed at his full recovery. Even his tiniest capillaries were as clean as those of a much younger man. Today, at age sixty-five, George no longer needs any pills. Needless to say, he is very grateful to have discovered Dr. Budwig's Formula in time.

LINSEED — PAST & PRESENT

THEN — Just what is this medicinal fat that forms the basis of Dr. Johanna Budwig's exclusive formula? You might be more familiar with linseed (Linum usitatissimum) as *flax*. Since prehistoric times, this graceful plant with its long, flat, elliptical seeds has been prized for its fibre, from which linen is made, and for the rich oil given up by its seeds.

Ayurvedic herbalists recognized the importance of linseed as a medicinal centuries ago. (*Ayurveda* is a very old Hindu system of natural medicine still practiced in some parts of Asia.) Herbologists consider the ripe oil-rich seeds of this botanical a superior internal demulcent (softening agent) and also use them in poultices for the treatment of rheumatism, gout, boils, and carbuncles. The oil is used as an enema to treat impacted feces. Mixed with lime water, the oil can be applied topically to promote the healing of skin lesions and to soothe the intolerable itch of eczema. The bark and leaves are believed to fight venereal diseases, especially gonorrhea.

The ancient Greeks and Romans used the brown, shiny seeds as a natural protein staple in their diet, and their ancestors followed suit as they spread across the entire European continent. The plant grows well in any temperate climate and was known in old India and parts of Russia, as well as South America and the early American colonies.

NOW — Linseed oil continues to be cultivated and is regarded as a high-quality vegetable oil in many parts of the world today, but most Americans look on it as merely an additive in oil-based paints or as livestock feed. In this country, the meal which remains after the oil is removed is compressed into cakes and used as a high-protein mineral-rich livestock food.

The central Europeans, in particular, value the healthful properties of this remarkable plant. Our cousins across the ocean can purchase *cold-pressed, virgin, unrefined raw linseed oil* as easily as we can purchase the over-processed, chemicalized and hydrogenated abominations that pass for vegetable oils lining the shelves of our local supermarkets.

THE OIL — Because the linseeds themselves contain from 33 to 43 percent oil, they give up their valuable liquid fat quite easily when compressed. When it hasn't been heated, filtered, and refined, the raw cold-processed linseed oil is a rich golden-yellow, amber, or brownish liquid. It thickens and becomes more viscous on exposure to air.

The light-colored refined variety which flows almost as easily as water, the only type of linseed oil available to the consumer currently in the U.S. (even in health food stores), has had all the valuable solid fats (the essential fatty acids the body requires) removed. Unfortunately, it cannot be considered an adequate substitute for the linseed oil we are discussing in this chapter.

RAW LINSEED OIL — In its *unrefined* form, linseed oil contains two important unsaturated fatty acids (linoleic and linolenic). When correctly processed, the oil consists of a healthy 58 percent essential fatty acids. These essential highly unsaturated fatty acids are converted in the body to *prostaglandins.*

In Europe, raw linseed oil is used therapeutically in the prevention and treatment of:

- **Cancer**
- **Arteriosclerosis** (reduces arteriosclerotic plaque/ cholesterol & triglyceride levels)
- **Strokes**
- **Cardiac Infarction**
- **Heartbeat** (irregular)
- **Red Blood Corpuscles** (maintains flexibility)
- **Liver** (fatty degeneration)
- **Lungs** (reduces bronchial spasms)

- **Intestines** (regulates activity)
- **Stomach Ulcers** (normalizes gastric juices)
- **Prostate** (hypertrophic)
- **Arthritis** (exerts a favorable influence)
- **Eczema** (assists all skin diseases)
- **Old Age** (improves many common afflictions)
- **Brain** (strengthens activity)
- **Immune Deficiency Syndromes** (cancer, multiple sclerosis, auto-immune illnesses)

Without essential fatty acids, prostaglandin biosynthesis cannot take place. The biological importance of prostaglandins lies in their high effectiveness, the range and diversity of their metabolic actions, and their wide distribution in the body. These chemically active substances affect the cardiovascular system, are present in the prostate gland, menstrual fluid, the brain, the lungs, the kidneys, the thymus gland, seminal fluid, and the pancreas. There are more than a dozen extremely important prostaglandins. All are derived from essential fatty acids. Without the essential fatty acids (present and active in raw linseed oil), the body cannot manufacture the prostaglandins it needs for healthy functioning. Considering the important part essential fatty acids play in manufacturing prostaglandins, it's easy to see why raw linseed oil is so therapeutically important.

WHO IS DR. JOHANNA BUDWIG?

As you learned in the previous chapter, it was Dr. Budwig who discovered that the right combination of essential fatty acids (potent and active in linseed oil) and sulphur-based proteins (present in abundance in low-fat cottage cheese) is the magic formula for conquering cancer and the other diseases of fatty degeneration. Dr. Johanna Budwig is known and highly respected around the world as Germany's premiere biochemist. In addition, Dr. Budwig holds a Ph.D. in Natural Science, has had medical training, and was schooled in pharmaceutical science, physics, botany and biology. In all courses, this brilliant scientist excelled. Here's how Dr. Budwig's momentous discovery came about:

Building on the early findings of her colleagues (as outlined in the previous chapter), three decades ago, Dr. Budwig began systematic research into the problems of fatty degeneration. The refinements in investigative medical techniques she needed for the type of analysis she envisioned were not available, so she developed them. Thanks to Dr. Budwig's pioneering efforts, the elements present in a single drop of blood can now be isolated and identified. She was on her way to solving the mysteries of fat metabolism and close to an incredible breakthrough in medical science.

Dr. Budwig began collecting and meticulously analyzing literally thousands of blood samples, both from healthy specimens and from the seriously ill. The data that she tabulated showed that blood of the seriously ill (including cancer patients, diabetics, those with precancerous conditions of the liver) was always, without exception, deficient in one of the important essential fatty acids (linoleic acid). Other deficiencies became apparent as well. Also missing were phosphatides (required for normal cell division), and albumin (a blood producing lipoprotein).

Without the normalizing phosphatides, cancer cells (an abnormality) grow wild and proliferate. Without albumin (a combination of linoleic acid and sulphur-based protein), blood analysis shows a strange chartreuse (greenish-yellow) substance in place of the healthy red oxygen-carrying hemoglobin that belongs there. This fact explains why cancer patients are weakened and anemic. Without linoleic acid, the body can't produce hemoglobin. Without hemoglobin, the blood is unable to carry vital oxygen to the suffocating cells and tissues. Energy production suffers; the cancer victim becomes progressively more and more anemic, sinks into lethargy, and finally dies.

The blood of a healthy person always contains sufficient quality protein and the essential fatty acids. Progressing from this point of fact, Dr. Budwig reasoned that the victims of the diseases of fatty degeneration could be restored to health by supplying a diet high in essential fatty acids and sulphur-based proteins.

To test her theory, Dr. Budwig determined to begin with the highest-quality oil available in all nature. With its rich content of linoleic and linolenic acids (both the essential fatty acids), the liquid gold of crude linseed oil fit that description perfectly. For the sulphur-based proteins, Dr. Budwig selected skim milk. (Note: The latest Budwig formula uses low-fat cottage cheese in place of skim milk). She fed seriously ill cancer patients a combination of 100 grams of skim milk proteins with 40 grams of fresh linseed oil. To make the mixture easier to blend (and swallow), she added 25 grams of milk. During the period of these early experiments, she drew blood and analyzed the samples constantly, looking closely for the most minute changes.

What she found was gratifying indeed. Over a period of approximately three months, tumors gradually receded. The strange greenish elements in the blood were replaced with healthy red blood cells as the phosphatides and lipoproteins almost miraculously reappeared. The anemia disappeared and life-energy was restored. Symptoms of cancer, liver dysfunction, and diabetes were completely alleviated. Today, after ten years of solid clinical application, Dr. Budwig's cottage cheese and linseed oil formula has been proven successful where many orthodox remedies have failed.

Because of the influence of the powerful oil processing industry in Germany (which continues to attempt to discredit her findings), she was denied publication in medical journals. Dr. Budwig has published her research on the properties and benefits of linseed oil under various titles, including *"Cancer — A Fat Problem," "The Death of the Tumour,"* and *"True Health Against Arteriosclerosis, Heart Infarction, & Cancer."* (Note: These books are available as German language editions only and are not published in English.) Dr. Budwig has assisted many seriously ill individuals, even those given up as terminal by orthodox medical practitioners, to regain their health through a simple regimen of nutrition. The basis of Dr. Budwig's program is the use of linseed oil blended with cottage cheese.

Because her research has been highly publicized in Europe, even the man on the street has long been aware of the dangers of consuming too much of the wrong kind of fat. To illustrate this point, Dr. Budwig tells a charming story published in the *London Daily Express* headlined "Fat In Your Frying Pan Can Kill."

A husband returning home from an exhausting day at work said to his wife, "Pan fry me a steak, dear, but throw the fat away." "Certainly, not!" replied his wife. "The fat I'll use to crisp your steak the way you like it cost 36 cents! Do you really want me to throw away 36 cents?" The husband, in mock horror, answered, "What! Your husband isn't worth 36 cents to you?"

Dr. Budwig teaches that the way in which the body metabolizes fat concerns every vital organ in the body, pointing out that people afflicted with liver and gallbladder problems in particular cannot tolerate fat. She also observes that a high-fat diet doesn't agree with any unhealthy person, but explains that the three-times unsaturated, oxygenated fats in linseed oil, when taken with protein-rich cottage cheese, are easily tolerated by anyone, even those seriously ill.

Dr. Budwig tells of giving a lecture in Switzerland to hundreds of people. As she was taking questions from the audience, a man and wife approached the podium and asked to tell the listeners of their experiences. Dr. Budwig passed the man the microphone. He told of his daughter who had a serious deterioration of one knee joint. Her doctors had said her condition was incurable, that medical science had no hope for her, that she would eventually be completely bedridden and, unable to care for herself, would require full-time nursing care in a sanitorium. The unfortunate young girl also suffered from a disfiguring case of psoriasis. The man said that he himself had a tumor in one lung and went on to tell of the health problems of his son. He then passed the microphone to his wife and she completed the story. She said that when she began insisting the entire family follow Dr. Budwig's recommendation to eat linseed oil with cottage cheese every day, gradually their health improved. She reported that all four members of the family regained complete and robust health on Dr. Budwig's simple regimen.

DR. JOHANNA BUDWIG SPEAKS

Dr. Budwig lectures all over Europe. Her fame precedes her and she is acclaimed on the continent for her important work. Thousands flock to hear her speak whenever she appears. The many people she has helped revere her and testify to the benefits of her simple program of health. During my recent trip to Europe in early 1986, I had the privilege of interviewing Dr. Budwig and learned first-hand of her exciting approach to the cure and treatment of cancer, heart infarction, arteriosclerosis, stroke, and other problems of fatty degeneration. I have spoken with Dr. Budwig at length, have studied her published research material, and read her many books with keen interest. We have had a wealth of her printed material translated into the English language and excerpt as follows:

"As far back as 1957, the Cancer Research Institute of Paris, France began studies to determine the exact differences between a cancer cell and a normal cell. As revealed during the International Congress of Nutrition, the French scientists announced that they had found a lot of undissolved fat deposited in the nucleus, body, and plasma of the cancer cell. In his book, *The Cancer Problem,* Professor Bauer of Germany said that fat can both dissolve tumors and cause tumors. Although at the time this statement appeared contradictory, we know now that there are many different types of fat.

"Following this line of reasoning, it is obvious that if we feed the body the highly unsaturated and oxygenated essential fatty acids it requires, along with the high quality protein which makes fat easily soluble, it will counteract toxic and poisonous accumulations in the tissues. If we also stay away from chemical preservatives, then many, many people will become healthy very fast — even some who have been given up by doctors and hospitalized to die. I have proved this premise many times.

117

"Every part of the body is affected adversely by the use of saturated fats, including the brain, the liver, the kidneys, and the nervous system. But the function of the heart is perhaps the hardest hit when a disturbance in the fat metabolism occurs. When the wrong kind of fat has been ingested, it is transported via the blood and lymph. Fat globules (atherosclerotic plaque) are deposited in these vital pathways leading to heart disease.

"Poor nutrition gives rise to many problems. For instance, I once visited a woman in Switzerland who was suffering from terminal cancer. As a mother, her main concern was not herself, but the health of her two children, a boy of 12 and girl of 14. Both were obese and looked ill. I gathered the little family together and spoke to them of the importance of eating correctly. The daughter said to me in a soft voice, 'What is this wonderful preparation that can make us all well?' I explained how to prepare a cottage cheese salad dressed with linseed oil and how it could benefit the entire household.

"On the whole, I blame the older generation for the generally poor health of so many. Foods are commonly overprocessed and chemical additives are used to extend the shelf life and make more money for the manufacturers. The wrong kinds of fats are used and they are not pure. Many sexual dysfunctions are caused because the body cannot metabolize these foods. Fortunately, many health problems can be easily remedied simply by correcting the diet.

"When I talk about my linseed oil/high-quality protein fare, it is nothing but a simple food which contains the most active fat known to me: linseed oil. In this form, the essential fatty acids are easily assimilated and made soluble in connection with essential amino acids (protein) in the form of cottage cheese. This is good-tasting and very palatable. It has been used in Europe for many years by hundreds of thousands of individuals.

"I tell you now that this simple food can inhibit the growth of tumors. By completely natural means, fat metabolism is stimulated and the size of the tumor actually decreases. Of course, it is better that you not wait until three or four doctors and several hospitals have told you that your tumor is incurable. Instead, regain maximum health by always using the best nutrition. In a very short period of time, even the most seriously ill person will feel better.

"Very often I go into hospitals and take home very seriously sick cancer patients who have been told they don't have long to live. The first improvement which encourages these sick people and their families is when they say things like: 'In the hospital, I couldn't urinate.' 'In the hospital, I couldn't have a bowel movement.' 'In the hospital, I couldn't clear the mucus from my throat.' Suddenly all those blockages clear and the system becomes activated again simply because the linseed oil and cottage cheese I give are rich in essential fatty acids and electrons which emulsify the blockages and remove them. Sick people tell me, 'I feel so much lighter and not dragged down and heavy any more.'

"We have to return to this immune biological way of eating. I have been to Japan, China, and even India attending many scientifically oriented symposiums and have connections with many researchers in this field. They all wonder the same thing: 'Why is it that the biological approach of treating disease is so often attacked by authorities in the orthodox medical field?' I myself have been to court many times to defend my beliefs. Fortunately, all courts ruled in my favor.

"What is it that I am doing? It's very simple. If any cancer patient comes to me, I just give them simple, natural nutrition. That's all. What can we learn from all this?

"First, we must restore correct nutrition. Fats, proteins, fruits, and vegetables are very important. But we have to be careful to take them in an unrefined and totally natural state, as nature intended.

"Second, we should be careful to avoid foods which have been contaminated with chemicals through processing or refining or treatment with antibiotics and growth hormones.

"To stay healthy and maintain all the vital functions of the body we absolutely must be able to metabolize fat efficiently. The continuing research on fat metabolism in connection with oxygenation, absorption, and assimilation of energy is of immense importance. If we are to survive in the western civilized world as a human being and a race, it's time to think about living our lives through sound biological principles.

"The secret of the wisdom of the universe is that science must conform with nature. Science and nature must work in harmony. Time is running out for all of us. We must begin to think and act and, most importantly, eat responsibly for the health and welfare of the race."

FATS AFFECT EVERY PART OF THE BODY

Dr. Budwig appears to have discovered one of the most important secrets of regaining or maintaining health. Consider: When we compare a healthy heart with one that has just suffered a heart attack, we find that the diseased heart is burdened with an accumulation of fat. A victim of arthritis carries excessive fatty deposits in his aching joints and muscles, but a healthy person does not. An organ attacked by cancer commonly shows an infiltration of yellowish-white fat globules with the appearance of tiny cauliflower-like rosettes.

The first visible symptom of cancer is the separation of lipids (fats) from the surrounding tissue. Saturated, hydrogenated, chemically hardened fats can actually act as chemical carcinogens within the body. Dr. Budwig's research indicates that the trouble begins when the protein-bound fats, normally present as free-flowing lipids in a live organism, become separated from their protein carriers and end up as unhealthy deposits in various parts of the body.

FATS ARE IMPORTANT — Science has proven that fats play an important part in the functioning of the entire body. Fats (lipids) are vital for all growth processes, renewal of cells, brain and nerve functions, even for the sensory organs (eyes and ears), and for the body's adjustment to heat, cold, and quick temperature changes. Our energy resources are based on lipid metabolism.

Each and every cell in this miracle we call the body is protectively covered with a sheath of fats. The cell body (plasma) is interlaced with little lipid veins, often called the 'nerves of the cell.' These lipid nerve-veins are the connection between the nucleus and the outer membrane. They influence the care and feeding of the cell and the process of normal cell division by the use of tiny electrical impulses. To function efficiently, cells require polyunsaturated live *electron-rich* lipids, present in abundance in crude linseed oil. Polyunsaturated fats greedily absorb proteins and oxygen. It is a docunented fact that many people suffer from an oxygen shortage simply because they are deficient in these oxygen-active lipids.

Lipids are only water-soluble and free-flowing when bound to protein, thus forming an electric counterpole to their protein carriers. This vitally important type of fat contains accumulated energy in its electron clouds. When high quality electron-rich fats are combined with proteins, the electrons are protected until the body requires energy. This energy source is fully and immediately available to the body on demand, as nature intended. These energy resources can be instantly mobilized and rushed into action as needed.

The presence of these important lipids can be compared to the capital (money reserves) of a corporation. Any type of growth or activity, whether that of a corporation or the human body, requires an expenditure of capital (money or energy). In the body, any activity (physical or mental) or growth factor (during pregnancy or the normal growing period from infant to adult, for example) requires the presence of electron-rich fats bound to proteins. All the cells, muscle masses, brain, nerves, organs, and lifestreams (blood and lymph) of the body need these electrically-charged, highly-active lipids. The demands on these energy reserves are enormous. Every breath we take, every muscle we move, every time the heart beats — even the automatic process of renewal and division of every cell in the body — depends on this energy source.

Let's examine the benefits accruing to the heart from electrically-charged lipids. There is an immediate harmonious interaction with the heart when the spent venous blood receives a healthy dose of lipids from the lymphatic system immediately before entering the heart. Inside the heart, the venous blood and lipids are mixed, creating a measurable electric current which regulates the action of the heart and sends impulses to the entire circulatory system. This blood, now charged by the electron-rich lipids, then flows to the lungs where it is charged with oxygen and pumped through the left ventricle into the aortas of the body. The vital life-sustaining pumping action of the heart itself depends on the electrical charge created by the lipids.

Some highly respected oncologists (cancer specialists) have pointed out that the bio-oxidation of the cell is seriously inhibited in a malignant tumor. As bio-oxidation decreases, fermentation metabolism of the cancerous cell increases. The antioxidants used in the chemically processed oils and margarines we put on the family table obstruct the bio-oxidation of every cell in the body. However, virgin linseed oil *(cold-processed, unrefined, and additive-free)* actually stimulates the bio-oxidation of cells and tissues and normalizes the important oxygenation processes throughout the organism.

The frequent successes which have been obtained in treatment with the essential fatty acids and the lipotropic effect' of essential amino acids brings us quickly to the realization that only a combination of essential proteins with essential fatty acids can bring about the full beneficial impact of these vital elements.

THE IMPORTANT FOODS — Many of the foods we commonly eat are lacking in both essential fatty acids and essential amino acids. The essential amino acids (proteins) are present in abundance in cottage cheese, buttermilk, hard cheeses, whole wheat, fish, and lean meats. The essential fatty acids the body hungers for are found in rich supply in crude, unrefined linseed oil, soy lecithin, egg yolks, and some vegetable oils. The problem, of course, with most commercially processed vegetable oils that stock the shelves of our supermarkets is that they are heated, refined, hydrogenated, and full of chemical preservatives. Because the essential fatty acids are particularly sensitive to heat and oxidation, margarines and processed vegetable oils no longer carry their content of essential fatty acids. (See Chapter 5.)

It is only when the body is well supplied with the essential fatty acids and essential amino acids in proper balance that the metabolic system can function as nature intends that it should. In the presence of these vital elements, healthy oxygenated blood courses richly throughout the entire organism to benefit every cell. When the essential fatty acids bind with the essential amino acids, the offspring of this happy marriage are called 'lipoproteids.' Healthy people have an abundance of lipoproteids, but it has been observed that diseased patients (including victims of cancer) have a much reduced level of lipoproteids in their blood, or none at all.

By comparing the body to a wood or coal burning stove, perhaps we can form an easily understood mental picture, albeit very simplified, of the workings of the body. Let's say that the stove has been overheated often, it has been fed the cheapest grade of coal, and its maintenance has been neglected for a long period of time. The body of the stove, the stovepipe, and the chimney become clogged with a dangerous residue that could flare into flames at any time, and which might very well burn down the house. We must clean away the deposits and feed the stove well-dried wood that burns cleanly without leaving a harmful residue.

The body which has been wrongly fed, poorly maintained, and neglected is in the same sad state as the abused stove. Harmful deposits and a residue of fats clog the inner workings of the body. By introducing the clean essential fatty acids present in linseed oil and the superior high quality proteins (amino acids) present in cottage cheese, the body immediately goes to work to rid itself of the deposits inhibiting its normal functioning. By continuing to feed the body with these good natural nutrients, soon the body becomes healthy again as nature intended.

Needless to say, after the body (or the stove) has been efficiently cleansed and is free of harmful deposits, we're certainly not going to return to the same old suspect foods that caused the problem in the first place. In order to stay well, the experts say that good dietary habits must be followed rigorously for a lifetime.

EXAMINING CHEMICALLY PROCESSED FATS — Dr. Johanna Budwig preaches against the use of what she calls 'pseudo' fats. In order to extend the shelf life, to provide the market with a visually attractive assortment of liquid and artificially hardened fats (margarines) — in short, to make money manufacturers use chemical processes that render their products harmful to the body. These fats may be marked 'polyunsaturated,' but they are damaging to the body all the same. If you doubt the truth of this statement, please go back and review Chapter 5 carefully.

The chemical processing of fats destroys the vital electron cloud, demonstrated in the foregoing material to be of immense importance to the functioning of every cell in the body. Once the electrons have been removed, these fats can no longer bind with oxygen and actually become an obstacle to the process of breathing. The heart, for instance, rejects these fats and they end up as inorganic fatty deposits on the heart muscle itself. As we pointed out earlier, a diseased heart and its aortas clearly show deposits of these worthless, electrically dead lipids.

Chemically processed fats are not water-soluble when bound to protein. They end up blocking circulation, damage heart action, inhibit cell renewal, and impede the free flow of blood and lymph fluids. The bio-electrical action in these areas slows down and may become completely paralyzed. The entire organism shows a measurable loss of the electrical energy which is replenished only by adding active lipids to the diet. These nutritional fats are truly vital for man and beast alike.

In recent years, scientists have coined the term 'fat intolerance' and deplore the damage done by fat degeneration. It's hard to believe that science hasn't discovered the root of the problem. The body rejects chemically processed fats because their composition has been changed so drastically from what nature intended that they are no longer able to fulfill their function in the organism, but instead cause untold damage to the body.

It is interesting to note that Russia outlawed the chemical saturation of fats for the purpose of causing them to harden artificially, as in the production of margarine, as long ago as 1902. Dr. Budwig explains that it is impossible to correct the damage done to lipids once they have been hardened into margarine just by adding some linoleic acid. In order to obtain a high level of linoleic acid, the manufacturers put in a chemical combination of ethyl and methyl esters, not the pure natural oil. Much research has documented the fact that this type of artificial linoleic acid does not combat the symptoms of an essential fatty acid deficiency in the body.

In direct contrast to the chemically produced fatty acids, consider what happens when just a minute quantity (one microgram) of linseed oil is introduced into the bloodstream of a cancer patient. Because the natural fatty acids present in crude linseed oil easily bind with oxygen and protein, the blood of the cancer patient improves within four to six hours. The activity of these natural lipids in the blood stream can actually be microscopically observed.

Fat damage is apparent in the heart, the liver, the arteries, and is clearly visible in malignant (and benign) tumors. The source of this degenerative damage lies in faulty nutrition, in the intake of the wrong kinds of fats. These findings have been substantiated by cancer researchers from twenty-nine NATO countries. Surely, no health-care practitioner, no scientist, and no thinking person can continue to ignore the facts. The essential electronically-charged fats that are found in abundance in natural linseed oil are crucially important to the health and functioning of the body.

Dr. Budwig herself teaches that the most favorable way to attack cancer at its roots is by removing all 'pseudo' fats from the diet and introducing the true nutrition of the natural medicinal fats present in linseed oil.

HIGH FAT CONSUMPTION — Are the citizens of the civilized world consuming too much of the wrong kind of fat? Statistics show that overall fat consumption is on the rise. Research conducted with laboratory animals has given us an important insight into one of the metabolic disorders arising from the overconsumption of saturated fats. Lab animals fed a diet high in saturated fats greedily consume as much as five to six times as much food (including fats) as animals fed a normal diet. Even more important, this study showed that when the animals were fed natural fats from linseeds, they consumed only about one-fifth of the fat and one-fifth of other foods in comparison with the group of animals fed saturated fats.

This experiment showed very graphically that 'cheap' fats are actually very expensive, both in terms of cost and in terms of health. In an effort to ingest the essential fatty acids their bodies craved, the lab animals ate five times as much of the commercially processed fats as did the animals supplied with the electron-rich active natural fats. This may very well be the explanation of just *why* our overall fat consumption is increasing. After all, the human body is not so very different from the body of an animal bred for laboratory research.

The health and well-being of the organism depends entirely on the type of nutrition consumed. Research has demonstrated that normal growth, healthy skin, glandular functions (liver, gall bladder, pancreas, stomach, intestines, prostate, lymph), are especially dependent on active fats. Glandular secretions are dependent on natural protein-reactive lipids. When chemically processed fats (protein and oxygen inactive) are consumed, there is a consequent inhibiting of all glandular activity within the system.

One of the first symptoms of faulty fat metabolism, easily observed by any of us, is a drying of the mucuous membranes of the nose and mouth. The dried-out mucuous membranes of the typical cancer patient, resulting in a sore, raspy voice, are caused when the glandular secretions are inhibited by the ingestion of chemically processed fats. Not so easily recognized, but just as harmful, is the drying effect exerted on the entire digestive and intestinal tract.

QUICK IMPROVEMENT — After only two weeks on the Johanna Budwig regimen of high quality protein and electron-rich linseed oil with its essential fats, the emaciated patient starts to gain weight consistently as his appetite returns. From being resigned to an early death, his feelings change to the joyous anticipation of recovery. An improvement in glandular and mucous secretions in all upper and lower body cavities, including improved intestinal functioning, can be observed in mere days, sometimes in just a few hours. Both asthma sufferers and those with cancer of the tongue have found quick and profound help.

Critical observers have tried to label this phenomenon as a psychotherapeutic (mind-induced) effect. However, Dr. Budwig points to her years of observation of psychologically impartial patients. These patients have testified to the truth of their own well-being and state their cures were accomplished by a simple change in diet. Dr. Budwig's patients want to talk about the so-called 'incurable' tumor which disappeared, the weakened and debilitated muscles which became firm, the seriously affected digestive system which was normalized after only a few days on her regimen, the painful and irregular menstrual periods which became normal, the most advanced case of cancer of the colon which healed. Dr. Budwig says that, as the internal functions of the body are normalized, even the smell of the patient's stool becomes less foul. Swelling and edema disappear as normal urination patterns are again established. The cancer patient begins to live again as he experiences the return of well-being. Very soon, he is free of pain without the use of strong medication or injections.

WORLD-WIDE RESEARCH

THE USE OF LINSEED OIL — Linseed oil is an edible polyunsaturated vegetable oil and is used in cooking in many parts of the world. It is very rich in essential polyunsaturated fats (linoleic and linolenic acids). Because these fatty acids are known to be essential to the body, many researchers around the world are investigating their properties and trying to determine the benefits of adding linseed oil to the diet. The current research coming out of Europe can benefit us all by pointing the way to both a preventive and therapeutic approach to many diseases. The results reported by various scientific authorities, excerpted below, are truly astounding.

GREAT BRITAIN — This very interesting study entitled *Changes in the Rumen Metabolism of Sheep Given Increasing Arounts of Linseed Oil in Their Diet* gives an indication of the function of linseed oil and how it can benefit the body.

We quote, "It appears that the lowering of the concentration of acetate in the rumen was not the result of decreased production, but rather increased utilization, such as one would expect if lipid synthesis increased. Linseed oil added to the diet did not depress VFA (volatile fatty acid) production, but actually increased it. Results confirmed that up to 25 grams of additional lipids could be synthesized by supplying linseed oil with the sheeps' diet."

A 'translation' follows. *Acetate* is a substance produced in the body when fats are not properly metabolized. However, when linseed oil was added to their diet, the contents of the sheeps' *rumen* (first stomach) showed that, even on this extremely high-fat feed, the *lipids* (fats) were being efficiently used.

POLAND — In a paper entitled *The Cytotoxic Action of Unsaturated Fatty acids on Cancer,* the Department of Pharmaceutical Technology of the Medical Academy, Wroclaw, Poland, announced: "The fatty acids isolated from linseed oil were found to exhibit a strong cytotoxic in vitro activity against Ehrlich ascites cancer cells with minimal cytotoxic effect on normal cells (leukocytes) of the peritoneal exudate in rabbits. The fatty acids from linseed oil (1000 g/ml after a 3 hour incubation) gave 100 percent dead carcinoma cells."

In plain English, the near-miraculous news is that the active elements of linseed oil exerted a *cytotoxic* (cell destroying) action against cancer cells *in vitro* (literally, in 'glass,' as in a test tube or lab dish), but bypassed healthy *leukocytes* (white blood cells).

POLAND — In yet another study, scientists working at the Institute of Pharmacology & Toxicology at the Medical Academy confirm that linoleic acid has anti-thrombotic (anti-clotting) effects in animals and man. This report concluded that, "Replacement of dietary saturated fatty acids by linoleic acid lowers the risk for myocardial infarction as well as cardio-vascular death rate. The cholesterol lowering effect of linoleic acid was clearly demonstrated."

GERMANY — From the Department of Pharmacology & Toxicology, Martin Luther University in Wittenberg, Germany, comes a research paper entitled *The Influence of a Linseed Oil Diet on Fatty Acid Patterns in Phospholipids & Thromboxane Formation in Platelets in Man.*

Interest in mounting this study developed due to the fact that Greenland Eskimos, who traditionally eat a diet high in EPA (known to increase the metabolism of fat), rarely suffer from heart disease. Building on the work of G. Hornstra (as published in Lancet, 1979), the bottom line is that this paper demonstrates that a diet rich in linseed oil can lower the risk of arterial thrombosis.

Noting that "A linseed oil diet is known as a 'prudent diet' in Germany," the scientists reported: "A diet of linseed oil (30 ml daily) for four weeks raised the content of linolenic acid by twofold, of EPA (eicosapentaenoic acid) by 150 percent, and of docosahexaenoic acid by 70 percent in the serum of volunteers. The human body seems capable of transforming linolenic acid into EPA. This change coincided with a significantly reduced production of platelet thromboxanes (clotting agents)."

INDIA — The Department of Medicine, Patna Medical College & Hospital, Patna, India, has released the results of a study entitled *Influence of Linseed Oil on Cholesterol-Induced Atherosclerosis in Rabbits.* Beginning with the premise that many researchers have shown that saturated fats increase the severity of atherosclerosis, the Indian doctors adminstered 25 g linseed oil with their feed to 36 albino rabbits for a period of 18 weeks.

At the close of the experiment, the animals were sacrificed and the researchers reported: "Atherosclerotic lesions were absent in group L (fed linseed oil), but the percentage of atherosclerotic lesions was significantly high in the control groups (not given linseed oil)."

It is important to note that in the group of animals given PUFA (polyunsaturated fatty acids) along with a cholesterol-inducing diet of saturated fats, a greater incidence of cholesterol buildup was noted. Of this statistic, the scientists say: "The hypercholesterolemic effect of (the combination of) saturated *and* unsaturated fat in rabbits fed cholesterol is caused by increased absorption and retention of cholesterol."

Does this mean that all polyunsaturated fats are not created equal? Apparently so. Linseed oil itself is a highly polyunsaturated fat, but did not contribute to a buildup of harmful cholesterol or atherosclerotic plaque.

AUSTRALIA — Coming to us from the Royal Perth Hospital of the University of Western Australia 'down under,' is a study entitled *An Inhibitory Effect of Dietary Polyunsaturated Fatty Acids (PUFAs) on Renin Secretion in the Isolated Perfused Rat Kidney.* In case you're confused, slowing down (inhibiting) the production of *renin,* is good. Renin is a protein that masquerades as an enzyme and acts as a powerful *vasoconstrictor* (compressing the veins and restricting the vital free flow of blood).

Excerpting from this paper: "After a four-week regimen of diets enriched with linseed oil, safflower oil, or saturated fat (providing 20 percent of the total daily energy intake), the animals fed linseed oil showed a significant fall in the proportion of arachidonic acid in renal phospholipids (kidney fats) and a reduction in urinary prostaglandin excretion. In comparison with the other dietary groups, linseed oil feeding also resulted in a consistently lower renal vascular tone. Results suggest that dietary enrichment with PUFAs may contribute to the lower blood pressures observed." In theory, it might be said that the superior effects of the linseed oil diet are related to increased vasodilator (vein expansion) activity.

Another study from the same source entitled *Dietary Modification of Platelet & Renal Prostaglandins* provides a clearer explanation of the lowered blood pressure readings observed, as follows: "Changes in renal (kidney) function and blood pressure control were reversed by restoring essential fatty acids to the diet. Dietary linseed oil caused the incorporation of linolenic acid into plasma and kidney lipids with a relatively minor reduction in arachidonic acid when compared to the hydrogenated coconut oil control. Diets rich in linoleic acid have also been shown to delay the onset of hypertension (high blood pressure).

"Prostaglandins are synthesized from arachidonic acid which, in turn, is produced from dietary linoleic acid.

Prostaglandins are involved in a number of blood pressure regulating mechanisms and have potent direct vascular effects. Significant changes in fatty acid and prostaglandin metabolism can be achieved with fat supplements of less than 40 percent of energy. Rats on an oil-rich diet showed an average lower blood pressure than animals on the standard diet."

FRANCE — The National Institute of Alimentary Research, Dijon Cedex, France, has published a report entitled *The Transference of Cyclic Monomeric Acids into the Milk of Rats Ingesting Thermopolymerized Linseed Oil.* The results of this study of pregnant and nursing female rats fed linseed oil interjects a cautionary note into the otherwise unblemished record of dietary linseed oil.

The researchers found that the administration of linseed oil (100 g of linseed oil thermopolymerized at 275 degrees centigrade per kilogram of feed) to female rats during the period of gestation and lactation caused the death of all young, either at birth or in the two weeks following birth. Rats on a regular commercial diet up to the day of littering gave birth to normal young. When these same females were given linseed oil in their diet during the nursing period, the young rats did not die, but their rate of growth was measurably slowed.

WARNING: Although the amount of linseed oil fed the female rats in this study was proportionately much greater than would normally be ingested by a pregnant woman supplementing her diet with this nutrient, the results of this important research certainly indicate that *a women who is (or suspects she might be) pregnant should not include linseed oil in her diet until after giving birth and weaning the child.*

AUSTRALIA — The Microbiology Department of the Royal Melbourne Hospital in Victoria, Australia published a paper in 1981 entitled *Anti-bacterial Activity of Hydrolysed Linseed Oil & Linolenic Acid Against Methicillin-Resistant Staphylococcus Aureus (MSRA).*

We quote: "Methicillin-resistant strains of Staphylococcus aureus, which are also resistant to most other anti-staphylococcal antibiotics, are currently causing a widespread epidemic of hospital-acquired infection in the State of Victoria. Patients who are colonized with MRSA appear to run a greater risk of infection after operative or other invasive procedures than do those who lack these strains.

"For many strains (of MRSA) at low concentrations of linolenic acid and hydrolysed linseed oil, there was a striking reduction in the size of the colonies. Our data show that MRSA are sensitive to hydrolysed linseed oil as well as linolenic acid. Preparations containing hydrolysed linseed oil may have a role in the eradication of the staphylococcal carrier state and could also be useful for prophylaxis, especially in debilitated patients."

Not only in Australia, but all over the world, the risk of contracting a staph infection while in a hospital is very real. This landmark report on the antibacterial effects of linseed oil (and linolenic acid) should be given world-wide attention.

AUSTRIA — The German publication *Research & Technology* (Forschung und Technik) recently reported on a three year study being conducted in Austria. Armed with a government grant, several Austrian biochemists and local teaching hospitals in the area have combined forces to investigate the properties of linseed oil against cancer.

Beginning with the basic research and fundamental data of Dr. Johanna Budwig, the Austrian scientists acclaimed Dr. Budwig's successful cures of cancer patients over the past ten years. Because linseed oil has been shown to inhibit the proliferation of malignant cells, these medical authorities are adding their voice to those who call this miracle oil "a glimmer of hope in the fight against cancer." This three-year study, already showing that the application of the highly unsaturated fats in linseed oil works against cancer, is proceeding as planned.

SOME HEARTWARMING STORIES

The foregoing reports of laboratory research scientifically document the benefits of linseed oil, but make very dry reading. On a personal level, the following stories are representative of the wonders that crude linseed oil combined with high quality protein can work in the lives of real people.

Coming out of Europe, and most especially stemming from the work of German biochemist Dr. Johanna Budwig, we hear astounding reports on the great benefits of simply adding linseed oil to the diet. Dr. Budwig reports that the essential fatty acids present in raw, cold-processed, unrefined linseed oil require a powerful supply of concentrated protein (amino acids) in order to efficiently metabolize in the body. Dr. Budwig's recommended regimen of using one tablespoon of raw, unrefined linseed oil drizzled over one-half cup of protein-rich cottage cheese (please select the low-fat variety) daily apparently works wonders. Read on.

MALIGNANT OSTEOMA — Magda W. tells her story in her own words: "I was told by the most expert doctors that I would have to be operated on to cut out the cancerous tumor that was causing a swelling under my eye. They explained that the size of the tumor was much greater inside and that there was very serious bone involvement. The malignancy was too far advanced to respond to radiation treatment. The doctors planned to remove considerable facial tissue and bone. I was afraid for my life, but being a young woman, couldn't bear the thought of such disfigurement.

"When I heard about Dr. Budwig's linseed oil and protein diet, I was skeptical but desperate for help. After four months on this regimen, the swelling under my left eye completely disappeared. The doctors at the University Hospital gave me many exhausting tests. One told me, 'If I didn't have your previous x-rays and medical history in front of me, I wouldn't believe that you had ever had cancer. There is hardly any indication of a tumor remaining.' I never thought that using Dr. Budwig's formula would be so successful. My whole family and I are very grateful."

BASAL CELL CARCINOMA — An elderly woman of 76 years of age, Mrs. Erika H., was afflicted with a somewhat slow-growing cancer on the tip of her nose which nevertheless was developing into a particularly ugly and disfiguring *rodent ulcer.* (A rodent ulcer is a gnawing cancer which eats through soft tissue and bone.) Because of Mrs. H.'s advanced age and the site of the cancer, her physician was understandably reluctant to operate and was attempting to treat her in the traditional manner.

Although Mrs. H. disliked being seen in public, a neighbor persuaded her to attend a lecture given by Dr. Johanna Budwig which was being held in a nearby town. After hearing Dr. Budwig speak, Mrs. H. began taking the linseed oil/cottage cheese combination religiously, adding a few cooking herbs from her kitchen garden to overcome the oily taste. She also applied linseed oil directly to the site of the cancer every evening before retiring. Very slowly, the affected tissue on the tip of her nose began to regenerate and eventually the ulcer healed. Mrs. H.'s physician credits modern medical techniques, but Mrs. H. herself believes with all her heart that Dr. Budwig's 'recipe for health' was responsible for her near-miraculous cure.

HODGKIN'S DISEASE — At the tender age of seven years, young Tommy G. was sent to the Children's Hospital where he was diagnosed as having Hodgkin's Disease. The child was operated on and underwent 24 radiation treatments, plus additional experimental therapies that the experts hoped would be of some small help. When Tommy failed to respond favorably to these heroic measures, he was discharged as incurable and sent home. His sorrowing parents were told his life expectancy was less than six months.

While in the hospital, Tommy had gone from a sturdy little boy into an emaciated and frail figure. His arms and legs were so thin that the outline of his bones were clearly visible. He had burns and scars on his neck, under both arms, and in his groin from the many radiation treatments he had undergone. His voice was hoarse and his breathing labored. After only a few weeks, this unfortunate youngster lost his ability to speak entirely. The ear, nose, and throat specialist the parents consulted told them that Tommy's vocal cords had been severely burned by the radiation treatments. He was admitted to the hospital again, this time to die.

The desperate parents contacted specialists all over the world, including Europe, Switzerland, and America. A famous newspaper took up Tommy's cause and ran editorials pleading for someone to come forth who could offer hope for the child's life. All the specialists who replied confirmed the cruel prognosis: There was no hope or help for Tommy. At this dark hour, the miracle the family had prayed for happened!

Tommy's mother told their story for the press: "A friend sent me a printed piece about one of Dr. Budwig's speeches. This material gave us hope and I contacted Dr. Budwig. I wanted to give my boy her diet in the hospital clinic, but the doctors told me they didn't have time for this special attention. We took Tommy home and started him on the diet ourselves. I kept in close touch with Dr. Budwig. In just five days, Tommy's breathing became normal for the first time in almost two years. Three weeks later, his voice came back. From this day on, Tommy began to feel good again. He went back to school, started swimming, and by winter, he was doing craft work. He will soon be twelve years old and is now a healthy, happy boy. Everyone who knows him says how well he looks."

Tommy's story didn't end there. At age 18, a studious young man and a good scholar, Tom began training for a professional career. He knows he owes his life to Dr. Budwig and thanks her daily in his prayers. According to his college professors, Thomas G. is showing great promise in his university work. His chosen future career, as well as his life and health, appear secure.

CARCINOMA OF THE STOMACH — When Mr. William Y. (42 years of age, husband and father of three) began suffering from chronic indigestion, he chalked it up to the stress of his job as a prominent officer of the local bank. He took over-the-counter antacid compounds to relieve his distress and ignored the problem. The condition persisted and his wife began urging him to see a doctor, but he stubbornly refused. He soon began vomiting half-digested food after eating and noticed streaks of blood in his stool after a bowel movement. Frightened and worried by these developments, Mr. Y. visited his doctor who immediately rushed him to the hospital for tests. His worst fears were realized when his doctor informed him that it appeared he had a malignant tumor growing in his digestive tract. Fortunately for Mr. Y., there was as yet no involvement of the lymph glands. (Because the lymph travels swiftly through the body, any involvement of the lymph nodes means that the malignancy can spread very quickly to other sites. In the case of lymph cancer, prognosis is extremely poor.)

Mr. Y. underwent an operation to surgically remove (excise) the cancerous growth, which appeared to be totally enclosed within its outer membrane. However, because of the possible danger of the blood stream carrying minute cancer cells to other parts of the body, Mr. Y. was placed on a program of advanced chemotherapy on an out-patient basis. He suffered all the classic side-effects of this toxic treatment, including violent vomiting and retching, progressive physical weakness, and almost complete loss of hair. The exhausted and nauseated Mr. Y. complained that the 'cure' was almost too terrible to bear.

Finally, a sympathetic friend brought Mrs. Y. some printed material which told in detail of the success of linseed oil and enriched protein in cases similar to that of her husband. The desperate wife and mother purchased some cottage cheese and a vial of raw, cold-processed, unrefined linseed oil and coaxed Mr. Y. to have it as his luncheon every day. Beginning by choking down just a few small spoonfuls daily, Mr. Y. progressed to the point where he was able to enjoy the entire amount. At this writing, Mr..Y. has returned to his employment as a bank officer and is once again able to support his family. He has completely regained his former robust health. As a preventive measure, the entire family now takes a salad of linseed oil and cottage cheese flavored with a variety of flavorful herbs daily.

OSTEOSCLEROTIC SARCOMA — When he was 16 years old, Keith O'B. was told by the Chief Surgeon of a prestigious hospital that it looked like only an amputation of his right leg could save his life. A biopsy of young Keith's tissue was taken, which verified the surgeon's initial diagnosis. He was immediately started on an intensive program of radiation treatments, but still no improvement was noted. This young high school track star said he would rather face death than lose his leg. The situation appeared hopeless. Keith's distraught parents consulted with the most eminent doctors they could locate in many areas, but all confirmed the frightening prognosis.

Only a meeting with Dr. Johanna Budwig and her words of hope stopped the planned amputation in time. After just two weeks on the Budwig formula, Keith was able to completely extend his right leg straight out for the first time in many months. A medical examination conducted two months later revealed that the swelling of Keith's involved leg had receded considerably and his blood count had returned to normal. Shortly after that, Keith's weight was stabilized and his general feeling of well-being was much improved. Within just three months of starting on the linseed oil/cottage cheese diet regimen, he was back in school. The family reports that the Budwig formula remains a part of their daily diet. The entire family, including Keith, is in excellent health.

HYPERTENSION — A harried and stressed criminal attorney of 47 years of age, Mr. Whitman W. was not surprised when his physician told him he was suffering from high blood pressure and would have to take prescribed medication for the rest of his life as he was risking collapse from a heart attack or stroke. Mr. W.'s doctor also advised him to take a vacation and take it easy in his professional life. Mr. W. laughed shortly and briefly outlined the important cases he had on his calendar that would require long days and longer nights of dedicated hard work and intense concentration. He continued working at his normal furious pace until he was faced with extreme exhaustion and could no longer ignore his health.

Mr. W. was finally forced to turn his case load over to a colleague. He checked into a renowned European health clinic and spa and prepared to take the rest he needed to renew himself. The director of this famous clinic was an advocate of linseed oil and insisted that the patients be served linseed oil and cottage cheese daily. The chef outdid himself to make the required portions tasty and used different herbs and seasonings every day. Mr. W. discovered that he looked forward to and actually relished his daily cottage cheese salad, but didn't understand just why it was 'required eating.' It was not until his blood pressure registered normal without medication that the director took him aside and explained the effects and benefits of using linseed oil with protein-rich cottage cheese. Mr. W. has incorporated this simple meal into his daily diet and now finds his tolerance to stress has been immeasurably enhanced. He no longer has hypertension and his doctor has said he has conquered the risk of suffering a sudden heart attack or paralyzing stroke.

ATHEROSCLEROSIS — A middle-aged construction worker of 50, Mr. Hank C., was told by his doctor that his serum cholesterol was registering at a very high level and he was in danger of developing an arterial blockage which could result in a stroke or serious heart attack. This nutritionally-oriented and enlightened doctor outlined the dietary changes he wanted Mr. C. to make in his eating habits and emphasized the importance of including linseed oil and cottage cheese on the menu every day. Mr. C. carried the instructions home to his wife and she immediately visited the local market, made the necessary purchases, and began serving the exact meals that the doctor had prescribed.

After two months of healthy eating, including a daily salad of cottage cheese dressed with linseed oil, the doctor was very pleased to find that Mr. C.'s dangerously high serum cholesterol level had been significantly lowered and pronounced him free of the imminent possibility of a blockage-induced heart seizure or sudden stroke.

BRAIN TUMOR — When Scotty A. experienced blurred vision, loss of balance and coordination, plus a complete shutdown of his bladder with the resulting pain and pressure of suppressed urine, he went to a nearby medical research center for a series of tests. The examination showed arachnoidal bleeding due to a brain tumor. (The arachnoidea is a delicate intermediate membrane which encloses the brain and spinal cord.)

Mr. A. was promptly admitted to the hospital, a catheter was fixed in place to empty his bladder continually, and chemotherapy treatment began immediately. Because of the location of the tumor, the doctors feared an operation would leave Mr. A. both paralyzed and without his mental faculties. During the course of treatment, Mr. A.'s condition worsened and his health deteriorated rapidly. His arms and legs became paralyzed and he couldn't hold any food on his stomach at all. No matter what he was fed, he vomited violently. Intravenous feeding was administered. The muscles controlling his eyes became paralyzed, leaving his eyes in an open fixed position. In order to keep the delicate eye mechanisms moistened, drops were administered around-the-clock. The medical doctors and scientists of the Research Center informed Mr. A. that he was beyond medical help. At his expressed wish, Mr. A. was discharged from the hospital and sent home to die in peace.

A Swiss friend came hurrying to his bedside bringing both comfort and hope in the form of Dr. Budwig's formula. Scotty A. was surprised to find that the few mouthfuls of the formula he was able to take stayed down. He writes: "Since I went on the Budwig regimen, the paralysis of my eyes, arms, and legs has receded daily. After only a short period of time, I was able to urinate normally. After eight weeks on the diet, I was able to walk unaided for the first time in months. My health improved so rapidly that I was soon able to return to my work part-time. Shortly after that, I was again examined at the Research Center and my reflexes were completely normal. The Budwig diet saved my life! Ten years later, I was given a thorough examination at the Center as a follow-up. My incredible recovery has been written up in many medical journals and I have become what they call a 'text-book case,' and all because of Dr. Johanna Budwig's simple diet."

FAULTY METABOLISM — A young up-and-coming career woman of 33, Miss Georgine A., had been taking thyroid medication for many years on the advice of her physician, but still found herself grossly overtired, easily irritated, and continually fighting a tendency to put on weight. This attractive young woman literally put herself on what was almost a starvation diet in an attempt to maintain a svelte figure. When she responded to what was a very real cry from her body for help and 'fell off her diet,' she gorged on saturated fats and sweets.

When this happened, she often cried herself to sleep at night and fasted the following day in an attempt to make up for what she called her 'indulgence' the day before.

What Miss. A viewed as a lack of will power and indulgence was actually an attempt by her body to stimulate her into supplying the essential fatty acids and complex carbohydrates it required for healthy metabolism. Where she went wrong was in supplying heavily saturated fats and sugary carbohydrates instead.

One day as she was eating a hasty lunch of cottage cheese at her desk, she was joined by a co-worker who was having the same little meal. The co-worker took a vial of linseed oil from her handbag and proceeded to lace her dish of cottage cheese with it. Knowing this friend to be one who never 'dieted,' Miss A. questioned her about this 'strange practice' and was thus introduced to Dr. Budwig's ideas. We are pleased to be able to tell you that Miss A. now makes one of her daily meals linseed oil and cottage cheese and says she 'never felt better' in her life. Her days of seesaw dieting are behind her; she has tremendous energy and is moving up quite steadily in her career.

THE LINSEED OIL DIET ACCORDING TO DR. JOHANNA BUDWIG

Dr. Budwig is very strict when prescribing nutritional therapy for her patients. For those of you who are in real need of this information, but unable to make a trip to Germany, we are providing an examination of Dr. Budwig's methods, as experienced by Jane D., a close family friend well-known to some of my European relatives.

To my knowledge, this is the first time this important information has been brought to the attention of the American public. I know first-hand of the documented successes Dr. Budwig has achieved in treating her patients, including some who were considered terminally ill by the orthodox medical community. However, it is not the intent of the author to persuade anyone to discontinue medical treatment.

FOR THE SERIOUSLY ILL

Because Janie D. was unable to keep food down, her treatment started with linseed oil (4 to 8.5 ounces) enemas of this miracle oil. After a few days on the enema regimen, Jane was taking 8 ounces of freshly ground linseed (flaxseed) mixed with raw honey,* the first food she had taken by mouth in some time. Jane was able to tolerate this mixture surprisingly easily. *(Note: The consumption of honey is not advised for diabetics. Because honey is an integral part of the diet Janie herself followed, diabetics are especially warned against taking honey [where indicated], until and unless the regimen is first approved and regulated by a doctor.)

According to Dr. Budwig herself, any seriously (or even moderately) ill person will benefit by taking ground linseed and honey. Jane was given this mixture for a few days until her digestion improved and she began to feel better. She was also allowed freshly made fruit juices *without any sugar.* Especially recommended are fresh vegetable juices (carrot or celery), plus apple juice. (If prepared juices are purchased, make sure there are no preservatives or chemical additives of any kind. If you have a good juicer, it's best to prepare your own juices at home so that you know exactly what's in them.)

Jane was told that it was very important that she take a warm drink three times daily. Herbal teas (such as peppermint or rose hips), are excellent and may be sweetened slightly with honey. Sugar is expressly forbidden. Grape juice can be used alone, or to sweeten other juices, when necessary. A small amount of regular tea may be taken in the morning (a.m. only).

THE ALTERNATIVE — OATMEAL MASH

Jane was soon able to tolerate the pure ground linseeds with honey mixture very well, but her family had a healthy alternative to fall back on when she was feeling particularly weak. Here's how Janie's family fixed the Oatmeal Mash, in accordance with Dr. Budwig's teaching:

Put 3 tablespoons of uncooked oatmeal in 4-6 ounces of cold water and bring to a boil. Add to this soft mash, 3 tablespoons of freshly ground linseed (flaxseed). Simmer briefly and allow to stand over very low heat for ten minutes. Remove the linseed mash from heat and strain. A little milk may be added if desired, which also benefits the digestion. This mixture is of high nutritive value.

To vary the taste of the linseed/oatmeal mash, Jane's family prepared it with several different healthy nutrients. Janie's favorites additions were: (1) Mix ¼ cup fresh carrot juice into the hot mash and take immediately. Carrot juice should be ingested as soon as it is prepared and not allowed to stand, or (2) You may stir in ¼ cup fresh orange juice, or (3) Stir in ¼ cup grape juice (red or white), or (4) Stir in 2 tablespoons of very finely grated apple.

THE STANDARD LINSEED OIL REGIMEN:

After a few days on the cleansing and building regimens as given in detail above, the next step for Jane was to proceed to the standard dietary program. Because of Janie's long-standing illness and seriously weakened condition, the family put her on the following hour-by-hour very strict nutritional program, highly recommended by a friend who was treated by Dr. Budwig:

At 7:00 am: On an empty stomach, Janie took 2-4 ounces of sauerkraut juice. Note: Sauerkraut juice has a high lactic acid content which enhances fat permeation, reduces congestion, and facilitates fat metabolism, thereby cleansing and flushing out blockages. It also aids the digestive process. Even those with a sensitive stomach benefit from the lactic acid content of sauerkraut juice and soon find that even raw vegetables are easily tolerated.

At 8:00 am: Before eating breakfast, Jane had 4-6 ounces of warm herb (or regular) tea. Next, she especially enjoyed the breakfast 'muesli' the family prepared for her, as follows: In a deep dish, layer in bowl in order given: (1) 3-4 tablespoons freshly ground linseed (flaxseed). (2) Add any fresh fruit in season (sliced or diced), and/or fresh fruit juice (without sugar or chemical additives), (3) Optional: Add a layer of any kind of ground nuts (except peanuts), (4) To 3-4 ounces of low-fat cottage cheese, add 1 teaspoon honey, 1-2 tablespoons linseed oil, 3 tablespoons raw milk, and blend together. It is important to use a blender or electric mixer so that the mixture becomes completely homogenized. (Add a little additional milk if necessary). Then, (5) Layer the cottage cheese/linseed oil mixture over the other ingredients in the bowl. For variety, you may add any of the following to the cottage cheese mixture: Bananas, lemon juice, orange juice (mixed 2 to 1), carob powder, coconut (unsweetened), vanilla, cinnamon, and so on. (We remind you again that diabetics should avoid the use of honey, unless specifically permitted its use by their doctor.)

Between 10 am to 11 am: As a mid-morning pick-me-up, Janie had 4-6 ounces fresh carrot juice. One half hour later, she choose from a selection of either radish juice, nettle juice (with lemon), celery juice or beet juice (mixed with apple juice).

12 noon (lunch): Just before lunch, Jane took 1 tablespoon freshly ground linseed (flaxseed) mixed with honey and 4-6 ounces of grape juice.

After fifteen minutes (12:15 pm): The first course of Janie's noon meal was a salad consisting of: Dandelion greens, watercress, celery tops, radish, sauerkraut, freshly ground horseradish (not made with vinegar), and green bell peppers. This delicious salad was topped with a mayonnaise made from cottage cheese, linseed oil, milk, fresh lemon, a little salt, mustard, pickles, garlic, plus fresh (or dried) herbs to taste, whipped to a creamy consistency in a blender.

At 12:30 pm: For the second 'course,' of her health-building luncheon, Jane was served a tasty bowl of fresh vegetables (choose your favorites) simmered in a little water with herbs, curry powder, or a little linseed oil for rich flavor. (This vegetable broth may also be seasoned separately with yeast flakes or bouillon.) Along with her veggies, Janie sometimes had buckwheat (cooked as for rice), brown rice, potatoes boiled in the jacket, or fresh mashed potatoes (made with a little milk and linseed oil). As Janie began to feel better, she craved a sweet. Her favorite desert was the layered cottage cheese/linseed oil fruit salad described above, with a little extra honey and natural vanilla added.

At 3:00 pm: Janie's mid-afternoon pick-me-up was one tablespoon of freshly ground linseed (flaxseed) with honey and 4-6 ounces of grape juice (unsweetened), or fresh pineapple juice.

At 3:30 pm: After a half an hour, she had an additional one to three tablespoons freshly ground linseed (flaxseed) with honey and three glasses (6 to 18 ounces total) of fresh cherry or blackberry juice.

At 6:00 pm: Janie's light evening meal consisted of one cup (6 ounces) of soup made of buckwheat cooked in vegetable broth, seasoned with a little linseed oil for good flavor and 1 teaspoon yeast flakes.

At 8:30 pm: Before she retired, Janie enjoyed 4-6 ounces grape juice with 1 tablespoon honey added.

I am very pleased to be able to report that Janie D. improved tremendously on this special diet. At the end of just two weeks on the complete program, her energy levels were so repaired that she was fussing at her family because she wanted to get out of bed and do things.

Today, just seven months later, Janie is again caring for her husband, her three children, and her household single-handed. Someone meeting this radiant woman for the first time wouldn't recognize her as the frail degenerated person she was less than a year ago! You'd better believe that Janie has the whole family enjoying a portion of cottage cheese dressed with linseed oil every day.

Note: It may seem as if this around-the-clock dietary program is overdone, but I assure you that run-down and debilitated individuals benefit immeasureably by eating the recommended foods as specified. The seriously (or even moderately) ill person needs to eat more often to rebuild and strengthen the body.

*Freshly ground linseed (flaxseed) and honey is an important part of the recommended diet. This nutritional supplement is sold already prepared abroad under the name of *Linomel,* but is not yet available in the U.S. However, the preparation can be made at home by purchasing whole linseeds (flaxseed) and putting them through a nut grinder before mixing the crushed seeds with raw honey. We stress (again) that diabetics should not take honey except on the approval of a doctor.

A SIMPLE SUGGESTION

It's hard to believe that simply supplying the body with a daily dose (one tablespoon) of raw, cold-processed, unrefined, virgin linseed oil with the good quality protein present in (one-half cup) low-fat cottage cheese can make such a vital difference in health, but the benefits of incorporating this simple meal into the diet are well documented and backed by sound research. The essential fatty acids (linoleic, linolenic) that the body requires for healthy functioning and efficient metabolism of lipids (fats) are present in natural abundance in this ancient botanical, recently rediscovered.

As you have read in the foregoing material, scientists all over the world are quite rightly singing the praises of *Linum usitatissimum:* linseed oil. You just might want to consider the possible health benefits of adding a linseed oil dressed, herb flavored, low-fat cottage cheese salad to your daily menu. Judging by the unprecedented results achieved in research, it must be said that dietary linseed oil has to be an extremely powerful natural preventive and unparalleled therapeutic treatment as well.

It always pains us to bring you important news of a medicinal or botanical that is not readily available in local stores. Correctly produced (raw, cold-processed, unrefined, virgin) linseed oil is difficult, if not nearly impossible, to obtain in the United States. The brand you want — *C-Leinomed*™ (Linomed) produced to retain all its vital health-promoting properties. Major health food stores should have *C-Leinomed*™ but if you can't locate this unrefined virgin linseed oil locally, please see the final chapter for the name of the U.S. distributor.

Chapter VII

The Dietary Delights of Linseed Oil

How To Enjoy The Miracle Fat

THE BASIC FORMULA

As a dietary supplement, I personally take 1 or 2 tablespoons of cold-processed, unrefined virgin linseed oil mixed with ½ to 1 cup of low-fat cottage cheese every day. Because of all the very strong evidence, it seems to me that this is the best 'preventive medicine' in the world to ward off the degenerative diseases.

HOW TO PREPARE A LINSEED OIL & COTTAGE CHEESE SALAD

To the basic formula given above, we add herbs, raw vegetables, or fruits to taste, exactly as recommended by Dr. Johanna Budwig. We mince the herbs finely (or crumble dried herbs), grate raw vegetables, dice or chop fruits, and whirl in a blender until well mixed. The use of a blender is strongly recommended to insure that the oil permeates the cottage cheese completely and that the salad is well-flavored with your favorite additions.

The use of a different variety of flavorings is recommended so as not to tire of this healthy mixture. Garlic and onions are very popular health-promoting additions. Try finely grated cucumbers and radishes with some chopped tomatoes and a crumbling of dill. A combination of grated carrots and minced onions is both tasty and healthy.

For a sensational naturally sweet salad, coarsely chop a tart-sweet apple, add a small handful of raisins, a sprinkling of cinnamon, and a dollop of (raw) honey to taste.

The idea is to experiment by adding your own favorite herbs, vegetables, and fruits to the basic linseed oil and cottage cheese formula to provide variety.

MY FAVORITE BREAKFAST 'MUESLI' (MIXTURE)

Before eating this delightful breakfast 'muesli,' we take a cup (4-6 ounces) of warm herb (or regular) tea, in accordance with the standard regimen.

Here's how we prepare the 'muesli.' In a deep bowl, layer (do not blend together) in order given: (1) 1 to 2 tablespoons freshly ground linseed blended with a little honey (optional). (2) Add any fresh fruit in season (sliced or diced), and/or canned fruits or juices (without sugar or chemical additives), (3) Optional: Add a layer of any kind of ground nuts (except peanuts), (4) Prepare *cream topping,* as follows: To 3-4 ounces of low-fat cottage cheese, add 1 teaspoon honey, 1 to 2 tablespoons linseed oil, 3 tablespoons low-fat milk, and blend together. (It is important to use a blender or electric mixer so that the mixture becomes completely homogenized. Add a little additional milk if necessary).

LOWFAT COTTAGE CHEESE
HONEY
LINSEED OIL/FLAXSEED OIL
C-LEINOMED (Brand name)
Unrefined

FRUIT
(Ground Nuts)
Optional

Freshly Ground
Linseed/Flaxseed

Then, (5) Spoon the cream topping mixture over the other ingredients in the bowl. Top with a sprinkling of nuts, chopped
fruits, spices, or herbs.

For variety, we may add just about anything we like to the
linseed oil/cottage cheese cream topping. Try bananas, lemon
juice and orange juice (mixed 2 to 1), your favorite fruit juice,
carob powder, coconut (unsweetened), vanilla, cinnamon, and
on and on.

My wife and I enjoy this special 'muesli' every day. Please
don't think you can eat it only for breakfast; it often serves as
a light luncheon or dinner for us. I have introduced our friends
to this delightful combination and we've had many favorable
comments, especially pertaining to an incredible rush of sustained energy and easy weight loss.

One of my favorite people is a rather elderly gentleman (age
75) who lives nearby. Over the last few years, I have watched
him with a great deal of sadness as he became frail and
stooped. He got around painfully by supporting himself with
a stout cane and it was apparent that he suffered greatly from
arthritis. I tried tactfully to advise him on the importance of
eating correctly, but he always laughed and wouldn't listen to
any serious conversation on the subject of his health.

We were chatting a few months ago about inconsequential
things when my wife called out the window to tell me that lunch
was ready. I coaxed him into joining us and introduced him
to the 'muesli.' He devoured a whole heaping dishful with
obvious pleasure. Since that time, I know for a fact that he
fixes himself a cottage cheese salad generously laced with this
liquid sunshine every day. His improvement has been gradual,
but he is improving. On many days, he leaves his stick at home
because he really doesn't need it anymore. His formerly sick
and waxy complexion has become pink with the glow of health
and he continually expresses his gratitude for the increased
well-being he is experiencing.

DRESSINGS FOR SALAD GREENS & RAW VEGETABLES

We eat a lot of salads fixed with a variety of greens (spinach

148

is a particular favorite) and slivered raw vegetables. I like variety, so we use many different homemade dressings. Here's a few suggestions to get you started. Beginning with the basic blend of 1 tablespoon of cold-processed, unrefined linseed oil mixed with ½ to 1 cup of low-fat cottage cheese, try the following mixtures: *Creamy Italian* — Add vinegar and Italian herbs to taste. This is not only delicious on crisp greens, but also delightful as a dip for raw vegetables. *Thousand Island* — Add a little lemon juice, a little tomato juice, chopped hard boiled egg, and dill pickle. You may add honey to taste if you like this dressing slightly sweet. *Poppyseed Sweet & Sour* — Add honey for the sweet and lemon juice for the sour. Spark with a little dijon mustard, sprinkle in a generous amount of poppyseeds and enjoy. Wonderful on both a fresh fruit salad or the traditional greens. *Russian Dressing* — Add honey and lemon juice (as above), plus tomato juice (to taste). *Green Goddess* — Mince cucumbers, spinach leaves, and a little parsley. Whirl into the basic mixture and season with dill. *Hot Stuff* — Add cayenne pepper, minced chile peppers, a finely diced red bell pepper, minced onion, and blend well. Refrigerate for at least one hour to allow the flavors to meld. A real party-pickup when served with crisp raw vegetables for dipping.

THE BREAD SPREADS

Linseed Oil Butter — Many health-food stores offer sesame butter, but linseed oil butter is healthier and tastes better, to my way of thinking. The recipe follows: First, put 100 grams of crude linseed oil in the freezer to chill thoroughly. Then gently heat 8 ounces of coconut oil to boiling. (Note: Natural coconut oil is available in most health food stores.) Add a mashed clove of garlic and a medium onion cut in quarters to the simmering coconut oil. When the garlic and onions turn transparent (but before they brown), remove them with a slotted spoon and discard. Allow the melted coconut oil to cool off, but before it firms up, pour it into the chilled linseed oil. Blend thoroughly and pop your linseed oil butter back into the freezer to harden.

The garlic and onions add the sulphur the body needs to efficiently protect and process the essential fatty acids present in the linseed oil, so they are important additions. If you wish, you may substitute oats, peppers, or buckwheat in the recipe to provide the organic sulphur, but the resulting butter will be very bland. In either case, you'll find your linseed oil butter spreads nicely and is nutritionally correct. It is many times better than butter from the dairy and at least a thousand times better for you than the artificially hardened chemically saturated mess of fat known as margarine.

Mayonnaise — For a quick and nutritious bread-spread, add a dab of milk to the basic mixture, season with a spicy salt-free blend of powdered herbs (the supermarket has several good ones), and homogenize completely in a blender. (One of my all-time favorite additions to this mayonnaise is horseradish, freshly grated if possible.)

THE MAIN MEAL

Any meal should begin with a portion of raw, uncooked foods. We like to start off with a mixed green and raw vegetable salad topped with one of the dressing recipes given earlier. We always add some shredded carrots in our salads for their rich content of beta-carotene. Or we sometimes begin the meal with a slice of melon or other fresh fruit. Next, we have a side dish of the basic linseed oil/cottage cheese mixture, well flavored with our favorite additions.

We often have a bowl of good homemade soup, such as lentil, barley, or pea, for some high-quality vegetable protein. Adding a fluffy baked potato alongside makes the meal particularly satisfying. We sometimes enjoy potatoes with linseed oil butter and powdered herbs and spices, but my personal favorite is fixed this way: I cut the hot potato in half (the long way); top it with a scoop of low-fat cottage cheese; drizzle on some golden linseed oil; add some raw sweet onion (finely minced), and then fork the topping mixture all through the tender meat of the potato. A sprinkling of paprika on top, and the common old spud is transformed into an epicurean delight.

THE SWEET FINALE

I can't help it. I have to finish off a meal with a bite of something sweet, but I don't have to feel guilty about it when that something sweet begins with the basic linseed oil and cottage cheese mixture. It's easy to add a handful of berries in season (or any other of Mother Nature's sweet fruits), a spoonful of honey (or a dab of maple syrup, sensational with minced apple), and some vanilla (cinnamon, nutmeg, cloves, allspice, mint). Stir in any chopped nuts (except peanuts) for a family delight — or top with some slivered almonds for an elegant 'company' dessert.

A FINAL NOTE

The beauty of it is that the golden healing nutrition of linseed oil and the sulphur-based proteins of low-fat cottage cheese which comprise the basic mixture are bland enough alone to lend themselves to just about any combination of flavors that you can come up with. The possibilities are virtually unlimited. Let your imagination be your guide. Have fun with it by providing variety — and let the dietary delights of this healthful healing combination of the essential fatty acids and quality proteins insure you and your family of vibrant health and vitality forever.

PROCEED WITH CAUTION — My enthusiasm for the nutritional gold of virgin linseed oil must be toned down with a word of advice. This liquid sunshine is incredibly rich in the essential fats which, as we have discovered to our sorrow, are usually deficient in the American diet. For this reason, those new to this way of eating should make haste slowly so as not to shock a system accustomed to chemically altered and refined foods. It is best to begin with only a scant teaspoon of linseed oil blended into one-half to one cup of low-fat cottage cheese daily for a period of a few days to allow your body to adjust. And I remind you again that diabetics should not use honey, except with permission of their doctor.

Chapter VIII

Golden Bee Pollen Is Real 'Health Insurance'

A Potent Cancer Preventive and Much More

In ancient China, natural healers were paid a monthly stipend to watch over a family. Their task was to keep all the family members well. These early physicians were regularly consulted on all matters pertaining to health, prescribed herbal preventives, scolded when an ill-advised action threatened the well being of one in their care, and generally practiced a very effective form of preventive medicine. If an individual in their charge fell ill, the monthly fee was not paid by the family until that person was returned to robust and glowing health. I call that true 'health insurance!' In direct contrast, consider that our modern doctors are not paid until we develop a sickness. But in the highly cultured and advanced civilization of China centuries ago, the physicians had a very real incentive to practice good preventive medicine. That miracle food from the beehive, bee pollen, is amazingly effective preventive medicine and it doesn't require a doctor's prescription either!

BEE POLLEN IS SUPERIOR PREVENTIVE MEDICINE — As did the physicians of old, the natural healers of today call bee pollen a very effective form of 'health insurance.' One of the most interesting things about bee pollen is that it *cannot*

152

be synthesized in a laboratory. Oh yes, bee pollen contains all the vitamins, minerals, amino acids (proteins), hormones, enzymes, carbohydrates, essential fatty acids, and trace elements known to be needed in human nutrition. But, as if that were not enough, Mother Nature (personified by the bee) adds a mysterious extra that has so far defied scientific analysis. In fact, some researchers believe it's this mysterious unidentifiable extra constituent which makes bee pollen the powerhouse nutrition that it is. It's important to note here that pollen collected mechanically directly from plants (sometimes called 'flower pollen') without the intervention of the bee is without this important extra factor.

Another one of nature's little mysteries is the fact that bee pollen contains a live electric charge. Dr. Eric H. Erickson, of the University of Wisconsin's Entomology Department, reports that when the worker bees leave the hive, they have a slightly negative or neutral electrical charge. But, upon returning to the hive with their pollen baskets loaded, the same bees register a positive charge of electricity as great as 1.5 volts. The live energized bee pollen they carry is also electrically charged.

Just what is this incredible natural substance? Pollen is the live male spore of all botanicals and is necessary for fertilization and growth of the species. Each microscopically tiny speck of this golden dust has the ability to reproduce. Bees unerringly select only the most powerful and potent pollens as food for the hive, another reason why bee pollen is superior to mechanically-collected pollen. Although the adult worker bees subsist on honey, the tiny larvae are fed bee pollen to insure a good start in life.

Because the Queen begins life as a larva exactly like any other bee destined to become a worker, it is an indisputable fact that her exclusive diet of royal jelly (produced from bee pollen) is what causes her to become a creature far superior to the workers of the hive. The theory that bee pollen contains a rejuvenating, health-promoting, and life-extending force is based on the fact that the Queen bee alone lives for five or six *years* on her royal diet of royal jelly (which the bees manufacture from pollen), while the worker bees who eat only honey live for merely a matter of weeks.

EXAMINING THE EVIDENCE

INCREASING THE LIFE SPAN — Who says so? The Queen bee, Noel Johnson (the 87-year old Gold Medal marathon runner who was born in 1899), and U.S. President Ronald Reagan (born in 1911, now age 75, and a well-publicized proponent of bee pollen), are not the only ones who acknowledge the power of pollen to extend life expectancy beyond the norm.

The countries behind the Iron Curtain have published considerable research on the beneficial effects of this near-perfect food. Professor Dr. Nikolai V. Tsitsin, U.S.S.R. botanist and biologist, investigated the lifestyle of the centenarians past 125 years of age living in the Caucasus mountains of upper Russia. He reported that many were beekeepers and the villagers all ate the sticky residue found on the bottom of the hives as one of their principal foods.

On analyzing this mass, Tsitsin found it to be almost pure bee pollen. After intensive research, he determined that including bee pollen in their regular diet was responsible in a large part for the incredible age these people attained. Tsitsin was also impressed with the quality of their lives in that all these people were actively working and in singularly good health in spite of their advanced age.

Working independently, the same conclusions were reached by other U.S.S.R. scientists as well. Dr. Naum P. Yoirich of the Soviet Academy summarizes his research in these words, "Bee pollen is one of the original treasure-houses of nutrition and medicine. *Long lives are attained by bee pollen users.* It contains every important substance necessary to life."

Perhaps even more important for those of us discovering bee pollen late in life is the statement made by the Far East Institute of the Soviet Union in Vladivostok. These scientists concluded their research report by saying, *"Bee pollen has regenerative properties for the body.* Bee pollen contains all the amino acids, mineral salts, vitamins, and enzymes in perfect proportion as needed by the organism."

As a further demonstration of bee pollen's powerful regenerating and rejuvenating effect, consider a paper coming out of Sarajevo, Yugoslavia. In a well-publicized study, Yugoslav researchers at the University of Sarajevo used oral bee pollen therapy on a group of impotent men. After a thirty day period, over half were documented as showing an increase in the production of sperm, probably because bee pollen's gonadatropic hormones act as a reproductive-gland stimulant.

AN OVERVIEW OF THE BENEFITS OF BEE POLLEN

There has been so much material published in just the past five years on bee pollen that it's difficult to bring you a full and complete condensation of the many, many benefits this super-rich and incredibly nutritious food offers.

AS A STOREHOUSE OF NUTRIENTS — Because the important part that the daily diet plays in keeping us well or making us sick has been well established, suffice it to say that any food which has been demonstrated to contain every element the body requires has to qualify as a super-food. Laboratory analysis of bee pollen confirms that it contains all the health-promoting live nutrients the body needs to sustain life itself.

What's more, bee pollen, the super-food, delivers these nutrients in perfectly balanced proportions. And, isn't it nice to know that Mother Nature has packaged it so superbly? You really don't have to take laboratory chemicals with your breakfast in order to get all the vitamins and minerals you need daily.

Dr. Alain Callais, Academie d'Agriculture, Paris, informs us that bee pollen is richer in essential protein than any animal source and says it contains more amino acids than beef, meat, eggs, or cheese of equal weight.

MEDICALLY SPEAKING

Centuries ago, Hippocrates said, "Let your food be your medicine; Let your medicine be your food." As a medicinal food, bee pollen scores high points again.

CANCER — As long ago as 1948, the Journal of the National Cancer Institute published results of a study conducted by Dr. William Robinson of the U.S.D.A. which determined that bee pollen contains an active anti-cancer element which has the power to slow the development of mammary tumors. Tumor growth increased in subjects in the control group not given bee pollen. Dr. Robinson concluded that bee pollen is a powerful cancer fighter and stated that "These experiments were based on the postulation that bee pollen contains an anti-carcinogenic principle which can be added to food."

Dr. Peter Hernuss, a practicing oncologist (cancer specialist) at the University of Vienna, reported a "noticeable decrease in the side-effects of radiation therapy" on women with uterine cancer when bee pollen was added to their diet. Hair loss, nausea and vomiting, loss of appetite, bladder and rectal inflammations, were greatly reduced in the women who took bee pollen during the course of their radiation therapy.

HEART HEALTH — A recent Polish study (May 1986) entitled "Effect of Pollen Extract on the Development of Experimental Atherosclerosis in Rabbits" conducted by a group of scientists at the Institute of Pharmacology & Toxicology, the Medical Academy (Szczecin, Poland) agrees with earlier research showing that the oral administration of pollen extract contributes significantly to the lowering of blood fat levels. In a group of lab animals fed a highly saturated fat diet, those protected by the addition of pollen extract were found to exhibit blood cholesterol levels reduced by 67 percent and liver cholesterol levels reduced by 45 percent.

The Polish scientists concluded that the oral administration of pollen extract significantly lowered serum lipid levels and modified lipid deposition in major arteries.

PROSTATE — A German/Swiss team of urologists reported that bee pollen ingestion proved most successful as a treatment of prostatitis and prevented the need for surgery in their study of over 170 men.

NATURAL ANTIBIOTIC — French scientists (Dr. Remy Chauvin, the Institute of Bee Culture, Paris, and Dr. E.

Lenormand, the Paris Child Preventatorium) report that bee pollen contains an extremely active natural antibiotic able to correct gastrointestinal tract functioning by destroying harmful bacteria.

British scientist Dr. G.J. Binding says, "Honeybee pollen provides an increased resistance to infection. It is a giant germ-killer in whose presence bacteria simply cannot exist."

THE BOTTOM LINE — In his popular book, *About Pollen,* author Carlson Wade sums it all up by saying, "The healing, rejuvenating and disease-fighting effects of this total nutrient are hard to believe, yet are fully documented. Aging, digestive upsets, prostate disease, sore throats, acne, fatigue, sexual problems, allergies, and a host of other problems have been successfully treated by the use of bee pollen."

THE ENDURANCE FOOD

WORLD-CLASS ATHLETES — Lasse Viren, the Finnish runner who took the gold in the 5000 and 10,000 meter events in both the 1972 and 1976 Olympic games says his speed and endurance come from bee pollen. The renowned Finnish coach, Antti Lananake, concurs. "Our studies," he says, "show bee pollen significantly improves the team's performance. Most of our athletes take a bee pollen food supplement.

Of all the running champions, the most famous is Steve Riddick, long called the "fastest man in the world." Riddick himself says, "After just two months on bee pollen, I felt as if my body shifted into a more powerful gear."

It took former U.S.S.R. Olympic track coach Remi Korchemny, now with the Pratt Institute in New York, to provide the answers. Korchemny mounted a two-year double-blind study with Pratt athletes, giving some bee pollen and some a placebo. His conclusions proved beyond doubt that bee pollen increased their crucial recovery time after stressed performance and enabled the athletes taking bee pollen to actually improve their performance the second time around.

Noel Johnson, the remarkable oldster who runs marathons at age 87 and who enjoys what he calls his "second lifetime" with the verve and zest of a young man, agrees. Johnson says,

"I'll be in better condition at 90 than I am today. I know now what you have to do to rebuild and keep your cells alive and I know what causes illness!"

FROM THE HIVE TO THE TABLE

How do we secure this potent rejuvenating and health-giving miracle food for ourselves? Bee pollen is harvested directly from the hive by means of a pollen-trap fitted with a smooth wire screen. In order to enter the hive, the worker bee must pass through the wire screen. It gently brushes off a portion of the pollen she has collected in her travels from flower to flower which then falls a few inches into a pollen drawer.

The beekeeper then periodically empties the drawer of its precious contents and *should* (some don't) refrigerate or freeze it to insure ultimate quality and freshness. When he has amassed a sufficient quantity, the beekeeper sells his bee pollen to one of several U.S. manufacturers for cleaning, processing, and packaging into product form.

CHOOSING THE RIGHT BEE POLLEN

We want to say a word here about quality bee pollens. If bee pollen is bee pollen, why not purchase the lowest priced product available? Well, my friends, while a rose by any other name may still smell as sweet, that premise does not apply when selecting a bee pollen source. There are good bee pollens that deliver a full measure of benefits and there are poor bee pollens. No matter what end product the manufacturer turns out, that product can only be as good as the bee pollen and other ingredients that went into its manufacture.

For instance, when you find bee pollen granules that are as hard as pebbles, you may be sure that they have been over-dried at a heat high enough to destroy all the vital enzymatic action and reduce the nutrient value. You can easily apply this test yourself when purchasing bee pollen in granular form, but what about a capsulized or tableted product? It's very easy for a manufacturer to start with the cheapest grade Spanish pollen, for example. Once the product has been processed into capsules or tablets, there's just no way to determine what bee pollen has been used as its base ingredient.

Therefore, it's very important that you know and can trust the source of your bee pollen. By all means, shun all foreign products, some of which have been contaminated with carbon tetrachloride, most of which are heated, and all of which are old by the time they reach our shores.

In judging only the U.S. packagers of raw granules, there's more than one good brand available. Touted as being from the clean, sunwashed high mountains and deserts of the West, one of the newest and best is *Desert Gold Crown*™ from Biowell Co. Biowell purchases their raw product from the same source as does The Montana Pollen & Herb Co., producers of *Montana Big Sky*™. Another excellent source of granules is the C C Pollen Co., packaging under the well-known name of *High Desert*®.

These companies supply a very high grade of blended bee pollens gathered exclusively in the clean mountains and high desert areas of the Western United States. Because no single-source pollen can supply a full complement of nutrients, a multi-source blend of bee pollens becomes obviously very important. In addition, these golden grains are harvested far from the environmental pollution that drifts over the cities, streets, and even the farms of the nation, assuring you of fresh, pure, uncontaminated bee pollen with all the goodness Mother Nature intended packed into each tiny granule. In fact, the virgin high deserts and mountains of the United States might just be some of the few places left in the world where man has not intruded with chemical fertilizers, insecticides, and other pollutants.

In addition, any excess moisture found in these harvests is removed with an exclusive cold process at around 70 degrees. Testing reveals that each golden grain delivered by Biowell (Desert Gold Crown™), Montana Pollen & Herb (Montana Big Sky™) and the C C Pollen Company is full enzyme active.

Note: Pollens collected in many areas require the application of heat to preserve them from molding. Excessive heat destroys the live, vital nutrients so neatly packed into each tiny grain and kills the vital enzyme activity, resulting in a 'dead' food.

If you prefer the convenience of a premeasured dose, a powerful bee pollen product in an incredibly potent and unique new formulation is being sold under the trademarked name of *Bee Pollemed Gold*™. Each capsule contains top quality bee pollen, Siberian Ginseng, and the herb Gotu Kola, all integrated into a base of pure Royal Jelly. These additional ingredients both potentiate and synergistically increase the activity of the bee pollen, as well as providing important benefits of their own.

To show you exactly *why* we believe *Bee Pollemed Gold*™ is the best bee pollen combination product available, let's examine the active principles of each of the additional ingredients separately without regard to the bee pollen itself.

Royal Jelly — Royal jelly is called the 'rejuvenation factor,' and with very good reason. Science now recognizes the power of royal jelly to transform a single larvae (identical in every way to her sister larva) into the royalty of the hive, the Queen Bee. Just exactly how this mysterious nutrient accomplishes this miracle is still unknown, but it is a documented fact that the Queen Bee lives for up to *five years,* while the worker bees of the hive have a lifespan of mere weeks. The only difference between the two is that the Queen alone feasts on royal jelly for the whole of her extended lifespan.

Can royal jelly work this same miracle in man? Research coming out of the U.S.S.R. confirms that royal jelly contains *acetylcholine,* an important element shown to be lacking in the brains of Alzheimer's Disease victims on autopsy. The Soviet findings also state that royal jelly regulates blood pressure, stimulates the suprarenal glands, enhances the immune system, is effective in cases of arteriosclerosis and coronary deficiency, reduces cholesterol, and restores energy where it is lacking.

Siberian Ginseng — In contrast to the more common Korean ginseng (grown strictly for the lucrative commercial market in worn out fields), Siberian ginseng (*Eleutherococcus*) is expensive, but worth it. It is biologically active, very potent, and possesses all the properties that have made ginseng sought after for centuries.

In the traditional Chinese pharmacopeia of medicines, ginseng is known as the cure-all herb. It contains Vitamins A, B12, and E, plus thiamine, riboflavin, niacin, calcium, iron, phosphorus, potassium, magnesium, and sulphur. Ginseng is used in the Orient to overcome stress, to stimulate and improve brain function, as an antidote to drugs and toxins, to normalize blood pressure, reduce harmful cholesterol levels, and to energize and generally enhance health. Ginseng is considered a powerful youth restorer and is said to inhibit the aging process itself. As a preventive, this 'King of Herbs,' has no peer.

Gotu Kola — Gotu Kola (Hydrocotyle asiatica) is a natural herb that comes to us from the exotic islands of the Indian Ocean where the native doctors believe it contains remarkable stimulating and rejuvenating properties similar to those of ginseng (see above). An ancient Singhalese proverb says of Gotu Kola, "Eat two leaves a day to keep old age away." It contains Vitamins A, G, and K, and is rich in magnesium, plus small amounts of Vitamins E and B, and certain minerals. Herbologists use Gotu Kola as a blood purifier, to fight physical and mental fatigue, and as a senility preventive.

Note: All the bee pollen products mentioned in this chapter are available in major health food stores nationwide, or may be ordered by mail direct from the distributor. Please see the final chapter for ordering information.

Chapter IX

An Introduction To The Macrobiotic Concept

The Yin & Yang Factors

In Oriental philosophy, the harmonious concept of *yin-yang* is depicted by a circle, with the light and dark half being equal. The yin-yang circle represents the universe and all that is in it.

The Yin-Yang Symbol

YIN — Yin is conceived of as Earth, female, dark, passive, and absorbent. Yin is present in even numbers, valleys and waters, and is represented by the tiger, the color orange, and a broken line.

YANG — Yang is conceived of as Heaven, male, light, active, and penetrating. Yang is present in odd numbers, in mountains, and is represented by the dragon, the color blue, and an unbroken line.

The significance of the yin-yang circle permeates every aspect of Chinese thought and influences astrology, divination, art, government, and even medicine. The human body, like matter in general, is made up of five elements: wood, fire, earth, metal, and water. Each of these elements is believed to be either yin or yang.

Controlling the proportions of yin and yang in the body is the basis of Chinese medicine. Chinese healers have used almost every conceivable natural substance therapeutically at one time or another to restore the balance of the yin and yang. The famous Chinese herbals from ancient times (over 1,000) were collected into one tremendous work, the *Pen-ts'ao kang-mu,* or Great Pharmacopoeia, by Li Shih-chen (1552-1578). This work totals 52 volumes and is still authoritative today.

Incidentally, a few of the better-known Chinese medicinals which have been adopted by Western civilization include: iron (anemia), castor oil (purge), kaolin (internal absorbent), aconite (an alkaloid pain reliever), camphor (relieves itching), chaulmoogra oil (leprosy), the herb *Mahuang,* which yields ephedrine (asthma) and the herb *Rauwolfia,* which yields reserpine (high blood pressure).

THE YIN-YANG THEORY

AN ANCIENT ORIENTAL PHILOSOPHY — In the body, oriental philosophy teaches that the two branches (ortho-sympathetic and para-sympathetic) of the nervous system are two halves of the same yin-yang circle. When all is well within the body, they work together in a complementary manner to control all the body's automatic functions. Illness and disease arise when the balance goes out of control. In the yin-yang theory, some sicknesses are caused by expansion (yin); some by contraction (yang).

For instance, a headache caused when the tissues and cells of the brain *contract* and press against each other is designated a *yang* sickness, while a headache caused by *expanding* tissues and cells pressing against each other is designated a *yin* sickness.

What happens because of an imbalance of the yin and yang factors can be seen very graphically when red blood cells are altered by placing them in different solutions. Red blood cells placed in water (yin) absorb the water, expand, and finally burst. Red blood cells placed in a concentrated saline (salt) solution (yang), contract, shrink and shrivel. But, in a solution of 0.9% salt, the yin and yang are balanced and the cells remain virtually unchanged.

THE YIN-YANG CANCER THEORY

IS IT YIN OR YANG? — As the yin and yang concept relates specifically to cancer, consider the medical treatment of breast and prostrate malignancies. Female hormones (yin) can control prostate (yang) cancer. Male hormones (yang) can control breast cancer (yin). When the two halves of the yin-yang circle are harmoniously balanced, the malignancy is brought under control.

The macrobiotic diet is a completely natural means of changing the quality of the blood and cells and bringing them into a harmonious and healthy yin-yang balance.

THE MACROBIOTIC CONCEPT

EXTENDING LONGEVITY — We find that the dictionary defines *macrobiotics* as the art of lengthening the lifespan, especially by a vegetarian diet. Therefore, in the strictest sense of the word, anyone eating only plant foods grown in the region where he lives is following a macrobiotic diet.

However, we are examining here the precise macrobiotic concept as espoused, refined, and taught by Michio Kushi. It is based on the theory that all degenerative diseases, including cancer, are the result of a way of life that is out of harmony with the universal order of things.

For instance, an examination of the length of our digestive tract and the structure of our teeth certainly indicates that whole grains, vegetables, and beans — all of which require long chewing and a lengthy digestive process — were meant to be the principal foods of mankind, with certain variations appropriate to peoples living in vastly differing climates.

In the tropical regions of the world, the people traditionally eat a diet of locally-grown vegetables and fruits, while in the polar regions, the people subsist almost entirely on a diet of animal products native to their part of the world. For most of the peoples of the world who live in a temperate climate, the principal foods have always been whole grains and beans, along with local vegetables and fruits.

A DIETARY IMBALANCE — The disharmony, leading to a dietary imbalance which gives rise to disease, occurs when we deviate from the universal order as it was in the beginning and eat foods which were not ordained for our climatic range. According to the macrobiotic theory, it is these foods which upset the delicate harmonious yin-yang balance of the body and create disease when consumed over a period of time.

THE RELATIONSHIP BETWEEN DIET & DISEASE — Because new cells can only be manufactured from the elements provided in our diet, inferior cells are produced by an inferior diet. As a cellular dysfunction, the macrobiotic system shows that cancer is a prime example of improper food consumption over a long period of time.

When our food intake consists of high-quality nutrients, we get rid of any toxins through the normal elimination systems of the body via urination, bowel movements, respiration and perspiration. If our intake becomes excessive, the body shifts into another gear and employs additional and more violent elimination techniques, such as vomiting, diarrhea, frequent bowel movements and/or urination, sneezing, coughing, or a flash fever.

Whenever I suffered from a bout of flu as a child with the typical uncomfortable symptoms of diarrhea and vomiting, my mother always said, "That's the bad coming out of you, dear." It's true. The body automatically attempts to expel mucus, toxins, foreign matter, and harmful bacteria by all means at its command.

For instance, the macrobiotic concept explains that a chronic skin condition (or disease) may indicate that the eliminative systems of the body are over-loaded with toxins and the blood is no longer being properly cleansed. The sudden appearance of freckles and dark spots indicate the attempt of the body to discharge sugars and excessive carbohydrates, while white patches indicate the attempt of the body to get rid of excessive dairy products.

Further, when the bloodstream is clogged with fats and oils, the pores, sweat glands, and hair follicles may become completely blocked, resulting in chronic hard, dry skin. Dry skin is usually viewed as a lack of fats in the diet, but more often the reverse is true. When the blood is loaded with fats, moisture cannot reach the surface of the skin and dry, itchy skin results.

THE RELATIONSHIP BETWEEN ELIMINATION & DISEASE — When the eliminative systems of the body become exhausted or are prevented from efficient functioning by internal deposits of mucus or fat, the stage is set for serious illness. If these harmful toxins are not dissolved and discharged, they will be deposited in various parts of the body.

Typical sites of fat and mucus accumulations include the sinuses, the inner ear, the lungs, the breasts, the reproductive organs of both men and women, and the kidneys. Early symptoms created by these deposits may seem to be as far apart as a sinus headache is from a vaginal discharge or inflamed prostate, but actually they all result from the same cause: a buildup of toxic trash which the eliminative systems cannot remove.

If these toxins cannot be discharged, the body will continue storehousing the excess wherever it can. If high-quality nutrients are not immediately supplied to nourish cells and tissues, the cells will continue degenerating and a malignancy will flourish. Once the vital organs are infiltrated, survival hangs in the balance.

Think of what your kitchen would look like if for some reason you were unable to take out the garbage. You'd probably stuff all the trash and refuse in one corner and pile it up until the mess threatened to tip over. Then you'd be forced to select another site and another and another until your kitchen became so disgusting that you'd move out. Obviously, we can't vacate our bodies and move to a clean house. The only way we can clean up the mess we've made of our insides is by eating a proper diet. The macrobiotic diet is designed to clean up the mess.

HARMONY WITH NATURE — The macrobiotic concept also advocates both physical and mental exercise, a proven medical precept. Physical activity is necessary to stimulate circulation of the blood and lymph in order to eliminate the toxins present in the stagnant fluids of the body. Activities which stimulate body and mind assist in the production of energy and invigorate the digestive and nervous systems of the body as well.

Another important factor of the macrobiotic system is the distinction made between the *medically terminal* and the *macrobiotically treatable*. Certain medical procedures, such as intensive chemotherapy or radiation, result in a loss of some (or all) of the body's self-healing abilities. Macrobiotics teaches that the patient who has received drastic medical treatment must first recover from the toxic effects of that treatment before the macrobiotic diet can be effective against the malignancy.

THE CLEAN WAY TO EAT

PERSONALIZED NUTRITION — The standard macrobiotic diet is designed to provide the perfect balance of nutrients required for healthy cells. Only by encouraging the proliferation of healthy cells can we hope to guard against the development of any disease, including cancer. Macrobiotic foods assist the elimination systems of the body to dissolve and remove the toxins, fats, and mucus which can clog cells and tissues, leading to disease.

Macrobiotic experts caution that the same nutrient program is not right for everyone. If you are interested in pursuing the macrobiotic way of life, we urge you to contact the East West Foundation headquarters, whose address and phone number are provided at the close of this chapter. You will be guided to a highly qualified macrobiotic advisor in your area who will adjust the standard diet to fit your particular needs.

THE BASIC MACROBIOTIC DIET — The standard macrobiotic diet program is based on whole grains, beans, and cooked vegetables, along with certain supplementary foods, beverages and oriental condiments.

GRAINS — Whole cereal grains, including brown rice, whole wheat, oats, rye, corn, barley, buckwheat, and millet, should total between 50 and 60 percent of every meal.

VEGETABLES — Recommended vegetables include cabbage (green and Chinese), carrots, dandelion, burdock root, turnips (with tops), onions, squash (butternut and Hubbard), cauliflower, Swiss chard, bok choy, radish (daikon and regular types), watercress, and any other locally grown vegetables.

Total intake of the specific vegetables as recommended above should comprise between 25 and 30 percent of the day's nutrients. Up to one-third of the vegetables may be taken raw in a salad, but macrobiotic authorities say that persons with certain types of cancer should limit their intake of raw foods. Consult your qualified macrobiotic advisor to find out what's right for you.

Note: — Vegetables with a high acid or fat content, such as tomatoes, eggplant, potatoes, asparagus, spinach, sweet potatoes, beets, zucchini, yams, avocados, and green and red peppers, have no place in the macrobiotic diet.

BEANS & SEA VEGETABLES — A good health-food store or a shop offering Oriental specialties can supply the recommended mineral-rich sea vegetables, such as hiziki, kombu, wakame seaweed, nori, dulse, and Irish moss. The recommended low-fat beans include chickpeas, lentils, and azuki beans. Approximately 5 to 10 percent of the daily intake may include these delicacies, usually served as a side-dish or added to soups.

SOUPS — One or two small bowls of soup, seasoned with *miso* or *tamari* soy sauce, may be enjoyed daily. Prepare with the recommended beans, vegetables, and whole grains. Wakame seaweed should always be included.

BEVERAGES — Approved beverages include room-temperature spring water, any of the cereal grain coffees, roasted brown rice tea, roasted barley tea, dandelion tea, and roasted *kukicha* (bancha twig) tea.

SUPPLEMENTARY FOODS — A person in good health is allowed a small amount of low-fat *white fish,* plus a little fresh or dried *locally-grown fruit,* once or twice weekly. As a *snack,* roasted seeds, grains, or beans lightly seasoned with tamari, are permitted occasionally.

SEASONINGS — Sea salt, miso, tamari soy sauce, gomasio (sesame salt), kombu or wakame (seaweed) powders, Tekka, and Umeboshi plums are all delicious oriental condiments with specific benefits.

Note: — These seasonings are used sparingly. It is especially important to note that they are either *recommended* or *prohibited,* depending on the yin-yang balance of the ingestor, another reason why it's important to consult a qualified macrobiotic advisor before embarking on this type of diet.

MACROBIOTIC FOOD PREPARATION

BALANCED NUTRITION — There are several basic techniques in macrobiotic cooking that must be learned. In brief, a macrobiotic diet comprises healthy nutrient-rich foods containing a balanced complement of nutrients simply prepared. In the basic preparation, foods are steamed with a very little water. If oil is used, only moderate amounts of high-quality sesame or corn oil are allowed. Condiments add interesting flavor and certain condiments afford additional health benefits.

It is best to attend macrobiotic cooking classes. Classes may be available in your area. Take advantage of the opportunity to sample various dishes to find out what they are supposed to taste like and learn how to duplicate the specific culinary delights at home which will bring your body back into balance.

EATING CLEAN — If you are accustomed to sweet sugary foods, greasy fatty foods, heavy protein foods, excessively spiced and salted foods, and/or the thrice daily consumption of dairy products, prepare for an adventure. Be aware that your over-stimulated taste buds have become dulled and clogged, along with the rest of your body.

You will probably find the clean macrobiotic diet bland and perhaps even tasteless in the beginning. If you are one of those misguided individuals who is actually proud to say, "I live to eat," and who stubbornly persists in overindulging in spite of the consequences, it's time to change your style.

The following pages outline a few inspiring and documented case histories of those who have embraced macrobiotics. These stories show very clearly the health benefits that the clean way to eat and live has brought into their lives.

Once you have made the decision to *"eat to live,"* contact the East West Foundation headquarters for the name and address of a branch in your area. All Foundation affiliates offer counseling services, cooking classes, and courses in the macrobiotic philosophy.

The East West Foundation
17 Station Street
Brookline, MA 02146
(617) 731-0564

The case histories that follow are adapted from material which first appeared in the *East West Journal,* address given above. (All rights reserved.) We extend special thanks to the *East West Journal* for permitting us to present this exceptionally strong empirical evidence of the undeniable power of the macrobiotic way of life.

DOCUMENTED MEDICAL EVIDENCE

MACROBIOTICS vs PROSTATE CANCER — In 1975, a gentleman in his mid-fifties, Mr. I.M., was diagnosed as suffering from prostate cancer and began conventional medical treatment. The disease spread into his spine, his right hip, and his right shoulder. Medical treatment included surgery in which a portion of one testicle was removed (a partial *orchiectomy*), radiation therapy, and chemotherapy. Mr. M. also took hormones orally. He was in continual pain and vomited violently for 12 hours after every round of chemotherapy. Understandably, he became very weak and feeble. In spite of these measures, Mr. M.'s health continued to deteriorate.

Near the end of 1980, Mr. M. absolutely refused further chemotherapy, but agreed to continue with the oral hormones. He consulted an M.D. who recommended macrobiotics and got him started correctly on the macrobiotic lifestyle. Almost immediately, his appetite improved and his energy began to come back. Just one month after beginning the macrobiotic diet, Mr. M. decided on his own to cut his hormone intake in half. Within six months, he was no longer in pain and felt so invigorated that he stopped taking the hormones entirely.

Mr. M. attributed his dramatic improvement entirely to macrobiotics. He decided to have a bone scan to confirm his feeling that the cancer was being conquered. Radiologists reading his x-rays found that there was an obvious shrinking and clearing evident in all previous sites of the malignancy. Expert oncologists had to agree that the hormone therapy alone could not have accounted for the reversal of the disease evident in Mr. M.'s diagnostic bone scan.

Mr. M. says, "I follow the macrobiotic way of life. I am totally convinced that we are what we eat and that we literally destroy our bodies with the poor quality of foods we consume. At age 60, I continue to work full time and also often spend evening hours doing work. I maintain a reasonable amount of exercise and look upon cancer as something we can overcome with diet and determination. Our amazing bodies can heal themselves if we furnish them with the proper nourishment and eliminate that which is harmful."

MACROBIOTICS vs CERVICAL CANCER — At the age of 27, Miss D.G., a Licensed Practical Nurse, was diagnosed as having cancer of the cervix. After several Pap smears and two biopsies, she was treated by a surgical procedure known as *conization* in which several layers of tissue were scraped away from all around the cervix. Unfortunately the cancer cells reappeared.

Because her doctor recommended she continue taking birth control pills, Miss G. decided to change doctors. As an LPN, Miss G. knew hormones could stimulate the growth of a malignancy. Her next doctor was more conservative and agreed to monitor her condition closely by taking Pap smears every three months. The smears continued to read positive.

On her own, Miss G. began making certain changes in her diet, eating less in general and reducing her intake of fats, refined foods, and chemically processed foods drastically. It was not until about a year later that she was introduced to macrobiotics. She embraced the macrobiotic regimen completely and discovered the principle of balance as emphasized in macrobiotic teachings.

After just six months on macrobiotics, Miss. G.'s Pap smears read negative. Her doctor termed it a "spontaneous remission," but she knew better. Miss G. says, "The only thing I changed was my diet! The conization hadn't worked. The cancer cells had appeared again after that had been done. Now, after 12 years, there has still been no sign of the cancer cells reappearing." The additional benefits Miss G. has experienced on the macrobiotic regimen are truly amazing. In addition to curing her cervical cancer, her hypoglycemia has disappeared; she no longer suffers monthly with PMS; the chronic lower back pain she experienced periodically no longer troubles her; the stuffed-up nose and blocked sinuses which had been with her since she was a child have cleared; her hemorrhoids disappeared; a psoriasis-type condition she suffered on her scalp and the acne pustules which were always with her are gone forever; she has lost a tendency to put on weight and reports her body has become more soft, feminine and graceful.

Miss G. says, "I would like to see nurses learn more about teaching patients what they can do for themselves, particularly in the area of macrobiotic, natural treatments. I think that nutrition and the link between diet and disease should become an integral part of nursing training. My own experience has shown me that this is just one more of the many wonderful things macrobiotics has to offer us today."

MACROBIOTICS vs OVARIAN CANCER — The doctors diagnosed chronic *endometriosis* (an infection of the lining of the uterus) and told Miss. T.G. that she would never be able to have children. Before she was twenty, Miss. G. underwent an operation to remove one ovary and a Fallopian tube. She was put on oral hormone therapy, causing her to lose all her hair.

Miss G. moved to another city and continued to suffer intermittent pain, which increased to the point that she went to a gynecologist. He determined that her endometriosis had flared up and also found a cyst the size of a small tennis ball. He recommended a complete hysterectomy, but Miss G. rebelled and moved into a macrobiotic study house. After just three months of clean macrobiotic eating, the cyst disappeared.

The attractive young woman's future husband took her to meet with Michio Kushi, the President of the East West Foundation. Miss G. says, "Michio could tell simply by looking at me that my left ovary had been removed and the remaining one was still very diseased. He also said I had a tumor growing in my descending colon and that I had jaundice. I was very inspired and convinced to follow the diet he recommended.

"For the next year, I ate very simply. Mentally, I was much improved. I became very meticulous about macrobiotics. Anytime I cheated, I would feel severe internal pain. As long as I continued with external treatments and the recommended diet, the pain would be nonexistent. One day I discharged a lump of cancerous tissue with my bowel movement. I began to feel much lighter as my intestines also improved."

Within a year, Miss G. married and the couple decided to have a baby. The pregnancy was easy and comfortable, as was the birth of a healthy son. Her second child followed a few years later with no complications, despite the prognosis of the medical doctors who had told her she would never be able to have children.

The happy young mother now says, "I know I was very arrogant and very sick. I had thought that macrobiotics would take the fun out of my life, but my life is much simpler and much more fulfilling than ever before. It's my sincere hope that many, many people will come to the macrobiotic way of life whether they are sick or not."

MACROBIOTICS vs WIDESPREAD CANCER — "You have a two percent chance of living out the year," the physicians bluntly told then 23 year old J.J. and his fiance, I.K. The cancer which had begun as a pea-sized lump on J.J.'s left testicle had spread into both lungs, his left kidney, and his neck.

After the complete surgical removal of his left testicle, J.J. was barely allowed time for his body to recover from the trauma of surgery before the prescribed chemotherapy treatments began. The routine was seven days of continuous treatment in the hospital, after which he was sent home to recoup and recover. When his blood count returned to normal, within two or three weeks, he had to return to the hospital for another bout of drugs.

J.J. suffered the typical side-effects of the chemotherapy, vomiting violently and spasmodically, and became weaker and more and more feeble. His condition was monitored constantly to determine the effects of the chemotherapy treatments, but the results were not encouraging. After the third series of treatments, the doctors recommended an experimental drug (*sis platinum*) be used in conjunction with the chemical treatments. After intravenous administration of the new drug, J.J. went into violent, racking convulsions. Of the experience, he says, "I felt as if I could just let go and die right there."

That night, he dreamed his mother (deceased) came to him and told him, "Go to St. Joseph's." St. Joseph's Oratory in Montreal, Canada is the home of Brother Andre, renowned for his healing miracles. Pilgrims to St. Joseph's travel the multitude of steps leading to the cathedral on the top of the mountain on their knees to show their humility and reverence. The dream made a powerful impression on J.J. and he felt compelled to go up St. Joseph's steps on his knees to pray for help.

When he was sent home from the hospital to recuperate, J.J. and his fiance discovered her mother was practicing macrobiotics for a lupus condition. This was their first introduction to this way of life. They purchased books and contacted their local East West Foundation for more information. Upon visiting the Foundation, J.J. was told of the diet he should follow.

The young couple felt the first stirrings of a faint hope, but it was time for J.J. to return to the hospital for another round of chemotherapy and sis platinum. Afterwards, the battery of tests showed that the tumors in his lungs were still present and the tumor in his neck had not changed. Although his blood tests had improved, the fact that the tumors were still present after such intense treatment was not considered a good sign.

J.J.'s teeth were extremely loose, his hair was gone, the membranes inside his mouth were encrusted with sores, he couldn't stop vomiting, and was barely able to walk across the room. It appeared to his loving fiancee that the treatment was worse than the disease and she finally asked him, "What do you want to die of, my love?" Together, they decided to begin macrobiotics. J.J. stopped all medical treatment, including chemotherapy, and never resumed it. He left the hospital determined to make a pilgrimage to St. Joseph's. His fiancee accompanied him.

As J.J. made the tortuous climb up the mountain steps on his knees, he prayed at each step for his relatives, ancestors, and friends who needed help, but not for himself. J.J. grew up with the strong belief that God knows what you need; you don't have to ask. With each step up, he experienced a warm feeling that he would practice macrobiotics, the tumors would disappear, and he would regain his health.

And so it happened.When the young couple returned home, they began studying macrobiotics and put the program into practice. Once he began the macrobiotic diet, J.J.'s strength returned quickly. After a year, blood tests showed no signs of cancer and the tumor in his neck had virtually disappeared. His wasted body was fleshed out with healthy muscle, his hair had grown back, and he was once again trim and fit. A very vital young man, J.J. himself says he feels better now than when he was playing high school football.

In J.J.'s case, a great number of factors came together to bring him back from the edge of the grave itself. He had the unswerving love of a very determined young woman who refused to give up; he had the good fortune to discover macrobiotics and the good sense to put into practice the macrobiotic program which restored his inner balance; and, perhaps most important of all, he had a deep and abiding faith in a powerful, loving God and a rare belief in miracles.

Chapter X
Visualization Therapy

Conquering Disease Through Positive Imagery

A DREAM OF PAST & FUTURE WONDERS — It is said that an ancient super-race once (or perhaps more than once) existed on Earth and will come yet again. Faint representations of what we like to believe were incredible beings still remain, now eroded, but deeply cut in cliff walls or chiseled into stone figures or painted on faded and chipped frescoes. If the old legends are to be believed, these humanoid creatures either descended from Mount Olympus or escaped from a cooling and dying star in the chariots of the gods, but (in our innermost hearts) we cling to the belief that there once existed an advanced and mystical people who were somehow privy to all the secrets of the universe.

These wondrous beings were forever young. The women were all meltingly beautiful and the men were all stalwart and handsome. Illness and disease and wars and financial hardship and every-day problems with the children (or the boss or a spouse) simply didn't exist for these fortunate creatures. They could not conceive of such horrors afflicting 'the immortals' (as they thought of themselves) and allowed these mundane concerns to be visited upon those of us who are mortals instead. And, guess what? We have meekly accepted all these horrors and taken them upon ourselves.

Let us assume for a moment that the ancient legends are true. That a mighty and invincible people, far more advanced than ourselves, once did walk among us on planet earth. What would it have been that set them so far above us? If we reject the idea that all-powerful gods and goddesses mysteriously endowed with mystical powers from on-high occasionally deign to visit us, and instead consider the possibility that humanoid creatures from another star system far ahead of us in knowledge just might have reached earth in the misty recesses of our collective past, the one thing that would have given them the edge is *mind power.*

THE GHOST IN THE MACHINE

THE BRAIN — The brain is a mass of gray nerve tissue protected from harm by the bony cage of the skull. It is the brain which regulates and coordinates the voluntary and involuntary systems of the entire body. Tiny electrical motor impulses work through the nervous system to transmit the appropriate message to specific glands and muscles to initiate a variety of activities. Blood circulation and breathing are regulated automatically through the cardiac, vasomotor, and respiratory reflex centers.

Medical science says the mind is: "An integration of the functions of the brain resulting in the ability to perceive surroundings, to have emotions, imagination, memory, and will, and to process information in an intelligent manner." (Taber's Cyclopedic Medical Dictionary) This is as good a working definition as any, but science still cannot open the skull, dissect the brain, and point to 'the mind.'

THE MIND — If we look upon the body as a machine, and the brain (and central nervous system) as the computer which programs and runs the machine, we still haven't recognized *the mind,* and it is the mind that makes the whole system work. Before the teachings of Sigmund Freud gained wide acceptance, most of us would have agreed that the idea of subconscious mental phenomena was impossible. But, since Freud opened the door, the power of the mind to affect the body has been demonstrated time and time again.

Since the dawn of time, mankind has attempted to define and put a label on the mind. In *The Concept of Mind,* (Barnes & Noble, NY) Gilbert Ryle called it: "The dogma of the Ghost in the Machine." Ryle says, "Minds are not in space, nor are their operations subject to mechanical laws. The workings of one's mind are not witnessable by other observers; its career is private."

It is a documented fact that a large portion (up to 90 percent) of the brain remains unused. This vast untapped power can be harnessed and put to work to accomplish many wonders. Stroke victims, with therapy, can often train their brains to use new pathways for speech and motor functions when the old ones have been destroyed. If a physician finds it possible to excise (cut out) a cancerous brain tumor and, in the doing, severs important sensory nerves, another portion of the brain may be able to take over. Considering these facts, it really shouldn't be surprising to learn that we can harness some of our unused *mind power* and use it to heal the body of cancer and other terrible diseases as well.

PROCEED WITH CAUTION — Although it is true that the mind possesses powers science can't explain, it would be unwise in the extreme to rely solely on the following visualization techniques and either put off seeing a qualified doctor or arbitrarily decide to discontinue medical treatment if you are under the care of a physician for any condition, especially cancer.

VISUALIZATION THERAPY

THE SIMONTON APPROACH — Dr. O. Carl Simonton (Cancer Counseling & Research Center, Dallas, Texas) explains that cancer, in particular, will flourish in a body whose owner is in a state of deep despair. Dr. Simonton says that psychological forces in the innermost recesses of the mind can actually assist the growth and development of a malignancy. On the other hand, Dr. Simonton teaches that psychological mind power can be consciously activated to battle and conquer disease.

After psychological testing and an intensive physical examination, Dr. Simonton puts his patients into psychotherapy.

During these sessions, he teaches his patients the technique of what he calls *imaging*. His patients learn to stimulate their immune-defense system by imagining a fierce internal battle proceeding in the area of their cancers, with the healthy cells conquering the malignant cells.

Dr. Simonton makes it clear that he has completely rejected orthodox medical treatment, including chemotherapy and radiation. Dr. Simonton healed himself of skin cancer on his nose over a period of one year. Although we have no case histories available, he cites statistics showing that patients under his care who practice his technique of imaging have up to twice the life expectancy that might be expected for their particular forms of cancer.

THE SALOV APPROACH — Leslie H. Salov, M.D. (Director of the Vision & Health Center, Whitewater, Wisconsin) is a very effective teacher of visualization therapy. He reports notable success with a toddler of four and one-half years afflicted with five *angiomas* (blood tumors) behind her left eyeball. (Children are particularly good candidates for visualization therapy because their minds are not cluttered with negatives.)

Just three days after little Sara's left eye first became red and swollen, the tumors had progressed to the point where her eyeball was forced out of its socket almost three-quarters of an inch. Sara's eyesight was deteriorating rapidly in that eye and medication prescribed by her ophthalmologist had to be discontinued because small hemorrhages in the eye occurred. It was apparent that the condition was extremely serious and Sara's parents were told that the eyeball would have to be removed along with the tumors. The rapidly growing tumors were constricting the optic nerve itself and stressing vital blood vessels.

When they learned of Dr. Savlov's program, Sara's parents took her to him immediately. The doctor sat the child on his knee and explained to her, very gently, in plain language exactly what her problem was, how the tumors were growing, and what would happen. He showed her pictures and took much time with the toddler to make sure she understood her condition. Dr. Savlov asked Sara to think about what was happening to her and then draw him a picture. The little girl said shyly that she would do that.

The following day, Sara's parents brought her back to Dr. Savlov and she gave him the crayoned picture she had drawn. The picture showed an eye with the tumors behind it. The eye had an angry face, but with her mother's help, Sara had printed 'I love you' and written her name below the phrase. Dr. Savlov was very pleased with her childish but clear understanding of her condition.

The next step was to teach Sara his technique of what he calls *visual imagery*. Dr. Savlov told Sara that her mother would give her a bucket and a small syringe filled with red water. Sara was instructed to look at the picture she had crayoned of her eye with the five tumors glaring out from behind it. As she squeezed the red water in spurts out of the syringe into the bucket, she was to imagine that the tumors were in the red water. As she squeezed, the bulb would become smaller and smaller as the water spurted out. Sara was told that the tumors behind her eye would also become smaller and smaller until they disappeared.

After just one month, Sara's protruding left eye had begun to resettle into its socket, showing that the tumors were being absorbed into her system. With continued visual imagery, by eleven months later, Sara's vision was almost normal and her pretty little face had lost its deformed look. She is now completely cured.

Dr. Savlov developed his particular visual imagery technique when he himself found he was losing his eyesight due to a severe degenerative condition. After being forced to retire from practice because of failing vision, Dr. Savlov heard of visualization therapy and began practicing it on himself at home. At first skeptical at what he thought of as totally outside the realm of science, he became convinced and a strong advocate of this type of treatment when he successfully restored seventy-five percent of his visual acuity.

THE RUDEMAN APPROACH — A Californian by the name of Sheldon Rudeman successfully healed himself of lung cancer. When his physician told him he had less than two years to live, Rudeman decided to prove the doctor wrong. He began an intensive program of visualization therapy on himself and, cured of the lung cancer that orthodox medicine said was his death sentence, became a visualization counsellor himself six years later — a full four healthy years after he was supposed to die of the disease.

Rudeman tells of a seven-year old boy suffering with advanced renal (kidney) cancer. He taught young Michael how to visualize the cancer as a monster invading his body and trying to destroy him. Mike drew pictures of the cancer monster and showed the forces of good attacking it. Rudeman asked Michael just how long it would take for the forces of good to conquer the cancer monster. Michael said the monster would be gone by the time he was eight years old, six months away.

In an interview when he was a normal active eleven year old boy and in what his doctor termed "full remission," Michael was asked how he destroyed the cancer monster. He said, "I just shot it up with glue!"

THE POWER OF POSITIVE IMAGERY

UNDERSTANDING THE SUBCONSCIOUS — Dr. Jonas Miller (Sarasota, Florida) says it is very important to be truthful with your subconscious. Dr. Miller tells the true story of a physician acquaintance to illustrate this point. This physician, the victim of a serious heart condition, made a tape recording saying "Every day in every way my heart is getting stronger and stronger." Every night he put the tape recorder under his pillow where these words were fed into his subconscious over and over while he slept. But one morning the doctor was found dead in his bed of a heart attack with the tape recorder still repeating its hopeful message time and time again.

Dr. Miller explains: "Never lie to your subconscious. Don't say you're well when you're sick. Don't say you're getting better when you're not, as the doctor was doing. He was not acknowledging his sickness and was trying to cover over a truth, but his subconscious knew better. If you make a statement which is untrue, your subconscious will know you're lying and won't follow through with the desired results."

According to Dr. Miller, who is also an ordained minister, the correct way to prepare your subconscious is to first recognize your illness, reject it, and then feed it a complete picture of robust good health. A woman with a cancerous growth on her face once came to Dr. Miller saying, "I've got this cancer and I need prayer." He instructed her to stop identifying with the malignancy and claiming it as her own, which she did by saying *"I've got this cancer,"* and instead to credit it to the devil. With perfect faith, the woman did as Dr. Miller instructed and the growth disappeared.

HOW TO PRACTICE VISUALIZATION THERAPY

GETTING STARTED ON YOUR OWN — If you are unable to find a doctor or counselor to prepare a scenario encompassing visualization techniques for you, you can develop your own. First, acknowledge your disease, but let your subconscious know that it is an unwelcome invader which should be eliminated. Imagine the 'good guys (the lymphocytes and macrophage cells of your immune system) attacking and defeating the 'bad guys' (the diseased or cancerous cells).

You might picture a white knight in shining armor hacking away at dragon tentacles, or a David aiming his slingshot unerringly at an ugly Goliath, or a faceless monster being vanquished by purity. First develop a mental image of your disease to give it reality and sketch it to reinforce your subconscious concept. Then picture the very epitome of good in any guise you may imagine and draw in the good image attacking the evil image. Don't worry if your artistic ability is zero. Whether you're using stick people or geometric shapes or what appears to be a mish-mash really doesn't matter. The idea of putting the images on paper is to impress your subconscious with the process it will then initiate in your body.

If you wish to add props, such as Sara's syringe of red water, to further reinforce and impress your subconscious, go ahead. In fact, if your imagination is a little rusty and you are having difficulty visualizing the healing process in the way you want it to proceed, adding props is a very good idea.

You might want to start with a very large 'monster' potato, for instance, and cut away many small slivers every day while visualizing an internal tumor being gradually reduced by a magic knife of pure gold. Because visualization therapy is not by any means an instantaneous cure, once the original potato has become smaller, start in on another of medium-size and continue the slicing away process day by day to reinforce your mental image of a tumor disappearing sliver by sliver.

Or you might want to do a series of daily drawings showing a huge mass of diseased cells being consumed bit by tiny bit day by day by a simple sunshine yellow pac-man cartoon shape. Your daily sketches should show the mass continually becoming less and less as you visualize the yellow pac-man gobbling away at the diseased mass within your body.

On the other hand, you might opt to relax in some quiet place and concentrate on running mental images through your mind depicting the conquering hero vanquishing the dread enemy. Simply directing your immune system to marshall its forces of lymphocytes and macrophages and sending them on a search and destroy mission is equally effective without any outside props as long as your visual images are strong, purposeful, and powerful.

TWO DAILY SESSIONS — Most authorities recommend practicing visualization for at least two twenty minute periods every day. During this time, you are directed to concentrate intensely on developing and sustaining mental images of your disease being gradually conquered and eliminated by strong forces of good. Once your mental images are strong, your subconscious will deliver these images to you at will. At odd times during the day, call up the images to reinforce the immune system and give it a boost. It's also a good idea to begin and close the day with a few additional minutes of powerful visualization so that your subconscious is continually kept aware of its role.

HOW LONG WILL IT TAKE? — Who knows? The success of visualization therapy is dependent on many factors, including the strength of your commitment and your ability to persuade your subconscious to direct the internal forces of the body to attack and conquer. It is not a recognized and universally accepted medical or scientific procedure, but a great many documented cures have been accomplished by this means. *Visualization therapy does work.* — If you decide to use this dynamic technique to eliminate disease and restore health in your life, let us know of your experiences. We care.

Chapter XI

Little-Known Cancer Preventatives & Some Avoidable Carcinogens

Controversial Findings From Around The World

In 1962, 170 persons in every 100,000 died of cancer. In 1982, the tally was 185 persons in every 100,000. On the surface, it appears that the incidence of cancer has gone up an alarming 9 percent in the last twenty years. But the American Cancer Society points out that it is the escalation of lung cancer rates (tied inescapably to a proportionate escalation in smoking) which has caused the increase. The ACS points out that the death rate for most other cancers remains approximately the same as it was in 1962. According to ACS projections, over one million Americans will be diagnosed as having some form of cancer in 1986.

Is that good enough? Dr. John C. Bailar doesn't think we've received sufficient value for our money. The well respected *New England Journal of Medicine* (May 1986) carried an article authored by Dr. John C. Bailar of the School of Public Health at Harvard. Dr. Bailar contends that we are losing the war against cancer and puts forth a recommendation that he believes will go a long way toward solving the problem. Dr. Bailar suggests that researchers concentrate instead on discovering ways to prevent the disease from occurring in the first place. He suggests that for every dollar spent on researching a cure, two dollars be spent on researching preventive measures. We agree. A preventive approach will certainly benefit all of us now living and may eliminate the spectre of cancer hanging heavy over the heads of future generations as well.

Researchers around the world have been coming up with some startling data. Although most of the findings from various parts of the globe regarding cancer preventives and/or cancer therapies are based on sound scientific theory and are founded on impressive clinical research, very little of this vital information has been made available to the American public until now.

LAETRILE—A CASE IN POINT

The name *Laetrile,* an apricot pit formula which was developed at the John Beard Memorial Foundation in San Francisco, is a registered trademark coined in 1952 by its discoverer, Ernst Krebs, Jr. Laetrile is a combination of the term *laevorotary* (having the ability to turn polarized light to the left) and *nitrile* (an organic compound in which nitrogen exists with all three of the displaced hydrogen atoms). Laetrile is commonly misused as a generic term for *amygdalin* (B-17).

AMYGDALIN — Amygdalin is found in over a thousand foods, one or more of which most of us eat every day. Lettuce, corn, kidney beans, sugar cane, millet, cassava, sorghum, lima beans, sweet potatoes and linseed all contain amygdalin. Strawberries, raspberries, blackberries, boysenberries, cranberries, elderberries, mulberries, gooseberries, huckleberries, loganberries and chokeberries furnish amygdalin. (Note: Amygdalin is more abundant in wild berries than in cultivated.) And, although we don't usually crunch the hard pits of the following popular fruits, amygdalin is also present in the seeds of apples, apricots, bitter almonds, cherries, peaches, plums, and prunes. (Note: Sweet almonds contain very little amygdalin.)

Amygdalin contains a natural cyanide compound which is not toxic in the human body and this natural form of cyanide is of immense value in cancer treatment. The malignant cell contains a special enzyme which releases the poison in amygdalin. The poison, in turn, attacks the malignant cell and assists in its destruction. Normal cells do not contain this special enzyme, do not release the cyanide, and therefore remain unchanged and unharmed.

When a correlation of data provides a comparison of people who ingest foods high in amygdalin versus those who do not, we may find an important clue to why some individuals contract cancer while others do not. If we are continually providing our body with foods containing amygdalin, known to attack and destroy cancer cells, how then can a malignancy grow and spread? Amygdalin will almost certainly prove to be an exceptionally efficient cancer-preventive.

The difference between amygdalin and Laetrile is that Laetrile contains amygdalin changed by a patented process from a glucoside to glucuronic acid. When amygdalin itself is ingested, either in foods or as an extracted compound, the conversion process from glucose to glucuronic acid takes place in the liver. Because Laetrile is already a glucuronic acid, the body does not have to initiate the conversion process. (Note: Extracted amygdalin is highly unstable in liquid form. Only dry, crystallized amygdalin is considered therapeutically active.)

Even though bitter almonds, probably the most abundant source of natural amygdalin, have been used in Chinese herbal medicine since 2800 B.C., the U.S. Food & Drug Administration does not consider the natural compound Laetrile a food, but has instead termed it a "drug." As the champion and sponsor of Laetrile, the McNaughton Foundation has handled all the red-tape and paper work necessary to bring this compound to the world.

After Phase I testing was completed by the FDA, Laetrile was pronounced nontoxic. By the end of 1978, more than 20 states had ruled that their citizens had a right to choose Laetrile as a holistic and nontoxic treatment for cancer and all seemed well. But approximately a year later, the National Cancer Institute filed an I.N.D. (Investigational New Drug) application and Phase II testing of Laetrile was scheduled. Phase II testing is allowed *only* after Phase I testing proves that the material being tested is not toxic in prescribed amounts. However, at a meeting of the Society of Clinical Oncology on April 30, 1981, Charles Moertel, M.D., of the prestigious Mayo Clinic announced, "Laetrile has been tested. It is not effective." Laetrile advocates believe that the Mayo Clinic test was faulty, but the bottom line is that this form of amygdalin is no longer legal in the U.S.

DATELINE EUROPE

Although the nutritional approach to treatment and prevention of cancer and the other degenerative diseases is rapidly gaining support in the U.S., our cousins across the ocean seem to be a step ahead of us.

GERMANY — One of the most comprehensive treatises on disease prevention and cure currently in publication is a scholarly work by the world-famous Hans Nieper, M.D. entitled *Revolution in Technology, Medicine, & Society*. Although this important book has been published in English as well as German, you won't find it in many local bookstores or even your neighborhood library. This work delves deeply into the causes of all the common diseases of civilization, including cancer, and explains some of the most successful methods of both treatment and prevention.

GENE-REPAIRING TREATMENT — Dr. Nieper says, "Some of the gene-repairing therapeutic measures for cancer, as well as protective measures for cancer, are already available and others will be added. Therapy should be applied immediately after the first discovery of, or operation on, a malignant tumor. This is mandatory. Any waiting game is fundamentally wrong. Modern gene-repairing therapy is practically nontoxic. It represents, so to speak, an imitation of the cancer defenses of the body. Today there is no longer any doubt about its high clinical value." In this chapter, we will briefly detail the findings, preventives, and treatments discussed in this serious work, plus outline the factors which are known to add to the risk of contracting cancer.

DIETARY CONSIDERATIONS

THE FOOD FACTOR — As a very graphic example of the chemical changes certain foods exert within the body, consider the case of a respected German physician which was presented at the Baden-Baden cancer congress last year. This physician used himself as an experimental tool to prove a point. After eating a meal of fried chicken, the doctor demonstrated that the malignant tumor in his neck was well-nourished and grew rapidly. In direct contrast, he found that a whole-grain diet of millet caused the tumor to be drastically reduced. In fact, the millet diet proved more effective in shrinking the tumor than orthodox chemotherapy.

This case alone proves that the body is influenced daily by nutrient intake. Diet plays a vital part in the *day-to-day* functioning of the body and does not merely affect the body over the long-term, as most authorities believe.

According to Dr. Nieper, the dietary recommendations of the U.S. Department of Health, Education & Welfare for a cancer-protective diet are incomplete in that there is no mention of the importance of Vitamins C and D2, magnesium, molybdenum, selenium, and beta-carotene in reducing the risk of contracting cancer.

OBESITY — Another factor which is stressed by knowledgeable oncologists is the importance of *under-eating*. Unfortunately, Americans are particularly fond of overeating. While an occasional holiday feast will not increase the long-term risk of developing cancer (as long as only the proper foods are enjoyed), carrying even a mere ten pounds over your ideal weight can add to your risk. A U.S. study conducted by Bayer Pharmaceuticals clearly showed that the incidence of cancer was reduced in laboratory mice especially bred to develop mammary cancer when they were consistently underfed. The healthiest exercise in the world still remains pushing yourself away from the table after a meager meal. Clearly, gluttony is one of the deadliest of the seven deadly sins.

Although German health authorities have not publicized a cancer-preventive diet, the recommendations contained in Dr. Nieper's book, *Revolution in Technology, Medicine, & Society,* follow. It is interesting to note that these recommendations are very similar to the recommendations of the U.S. National Research Council.

PREFERRED FOODS
- Whole grains (favored grains are oatmeal and millet)
- Skim Milk
- Fish (in limited quantity)
- Fruit and Fiber-Rich Vegetables (cooked and raw)
- Carrot Juice (freshly prepared)
- Pancreatic Enzyme Supplements
- *Omniflora** capsules and *Eupalan** bifidum flora containing milk
  (* German preparations)

RESTRICTED FOODS
- No Meat; No Sausage (6 or 7 ounces meat per week is permitted in cases of exhaustion, lack of blood protein, or cachexia)
- Little Cheese
- Very Little Sugar
- Very Little Fast-Release (refined) Carbohydrates (pastries, puddings, manufactured sweets)
- No Shellfish (because of its high nuclein content)
- No Smoking (or tobacco in any form)
- No 'Junk' Beverages (carbonated sodas, etc.)
- No Apple Juice (too high in glucose)
- No Distilled Water

Some of the most important anti-cancer nutrients targeted in this serious work follow, along with an explanation of the work they perform within the body.

BETA-CAROTENE — This important element is a *precursor* of Vitamin A. In other words, the body uses beta-carotene to manufacture Vitamin A. Unlike Vitamin A, research has shown that beta-carotene does not harm the liver. With their important content of beta-carotene, new research indicates that carrots may have preventive and even curative powers in the case of cancer, particularly of the lungs. The cancer-preventive properties of beta-carotene are stronger than those of Vitamin A itself. The powerful difference between the two is that beta-carotene carries a mysterious type of live electrical charge, while Vitamin A does not. Another important difference is that beta-carotene has little harmful effect on the liver.

As both a preventive and an active cancer treatment, beta-carotene has been shown to effectively destroy the cancer cell's protective layer of mucus, opening it to the body's natural defense mechanisms. Proponents of beta-carotene predict reductions in the rate of certain forms of cancer for those who regularly include carrots in their diet (up to 80 percent of cancer in the lungs and bronchia, and up to 55 percent in cancer of the colon). Carrots are the single most important source of beta-carotene in nature. This common garden vegetable is considered the first line of defense as a cancer preventive of the highest order.

It is important to note that beta-carotene is fat-soluble and can only be absorbed and assimilated by the body in the presence of a fatty emulsion. The essential fatty acids the body requires are present in trace amounts in butter and cream, but a daily regimen which includes linseed oil and cottage cheese may be a healthier way to ingest these fats. (See Chapter 6.)

Raw carrot juice is considered a natural solvent for all ulcerous and cancerous conditions. Many naturopathic doctors suggest that smokers and those with a family history of cancer may benefit by adding a cup of raw carrots or freshly squeezed carrot juice to their daily diet. Some authorities believe the preventive powers of this dietary supplement may also apply to ulcers.

SKIN DISCOLORATION — It is not the beta-carotene or the orange coloring of carrots which tints the skin. You don't turn 'green' after eating green vegetables or 'red' after eating beets or 'orange' after eating carrots (or squash or apricots). An intensive treatment with carrots may tend to impart a yellowish-orange tint to the skin. If this happens to you, rejoice! The condition is temporary and shows that so many toxins are being leached out of the body that the overflow is being released through the pores of the skin.

The elements in carrots assist in detoxifying and cleansing the liver, one of the body's most important organs. If the normal eliminative passageways (intestines and urinary tract) are insufficient to carry it all away, the remainder is released through the skin. As a matter of fact, the skin itself is the largest eliminative organ of the body. (The wonders of beta-carotene are also targeted in Chapter 4.)

CHOLINE & METHIONINE — Laboratory studies confirm that a diet deficient in choline and methionine fosters the development of liver cancer. (A.K. Ghoshal and E. Farber: "The Induction of Resistant Hepatocytes during Initiation of Liver Carcinogenesis with Chemicals in Rats Fed a Choline-Deficient Methionine-Low Diet," *Carcinogenesis* Volume 4:801-804, 1983). In this landmark experiment, the researchers fed young, healthy male rats a diet (peanut meal and soya protein) which was low in choline and methionine for up to two years. Of the 45 rats fed the deficient diet, over half exhibited liver cancer (hepatocellular carcinoma). In startling contrast, not one of the rats in the control group given a choline supplement developed cancer. The scientists noted that liver cell necrosis began within just four to five *days* after feeding the deficient diet, followed by a period of very rapid hepatocyte (liver cancer cell) proliferation.

This effect was noted as long ago as 1961 by I.C. Wells and C.N. Remy. ("Inhibition of De Novo Choline Biosynthesis by 2-Amino-2-methyl-1-propanol," *Arch Biochemistry Biophysics*

Volume 95: 389-399, 1961.) Wells and Remy showed that inhibiting choline synthesis fostered the development of cancer. A diet deficient in choline and methionine (dietary methyl) clearly predisposes animals to liver cancer, even when an external cancer-producing agent is not present.

However, because a choline/methionine deficiency produces free radicals which damage DNA over the long-term, further tests are necessary to find out if the increased incidence of cancer exhibited by animals on a choline/methionine deficient diet is caused by the deficiency itself or by the damaged DNA.

GARLIC — As a cancer-fighter, garlic has shown amazing properties. Building on early studies which showed that malignant cells did not produce cancer when injected into laboratory animals — *if the tumor cells were first saturated with an active garlic extract* — Japanese scientists have injected mice with an anti-cancer vaccine consisting of live tumor cells soaked in garlic extract. Fourteen days after the mice were 'vaccinated' against cancer, the researchers injected the mice with live cancer cells. Not one mouse died and not one developed a malignancy. In contrast, the mice which served as the control group (which were not protected with the garlic-based anti-cancer vaccine) all developed cancer on schedule and all died within a 30-day period.

Dr. Mei Xing of the Shandong Medical College (Shandong, China) says that the regular consumption of garlic can lower the incidence of stomach cancer by inhibiting the formation of nitrites and nitrosamines, known to cause cancer in animals. In his 1981 study, Dr. Xing determined that the human volunteers involved in his research who took just one-third ounce of garlic showed significantly reduced nitrite levels within just four hours of ingestion. He says, "My study shows that garlic reduces the concentration of nitrite in the human stomach and may thus be considered a protective factor against the development of stomach (gastric) cancers."

Garlic has been used effectively by healers for over 5,000 years. History tells us that the ancients had a special regard for the health-promoting properties of this pungent herb. The scientists of today confirm that garlic has antiseptic, antibacterial, antifungal, and bacteriostatic properties. Modern researchers name garlic an amazing natural remedy for some forms of heart-disease, high blood pressure, diabetes, dysentery, pneumonia, and yeast infections. Regular use improves the immune system, normalizes the metabolic rate (thereby assisting in a weight-loss program), and promotes high energy levels.

SELENIUM — Selenium is an important element currently under investigation around the world as a possible aid to a healthy heart. Many heart patients who have fallen victim to a cardiac arrest or cardiac infarction have been shown to be deficient in selenium. Respected authorities believe selenium affords strong protection against cancer as well.

However, it has become difficult to take in enough selenium in the average diet. Soil studies show that many food-producing areas of the world lack selenium in their growing fields. If the nutrient is not available in the soil, it cannot be present in the food. A selenium deficiency is very common among the populations of the civilized world.

MAGNESIUM — A 10-year long German study has shown that patients taking magnesium (aspartate and orotate) therapy for heart disease have a 20 percent less incidence of cancer than occurs in the normal population mix. This research validates the observation that in regions where the drinking water is high in magnesium, there is a much lower rate of both cancer and heart disease.

Magnesium is known to enrich the body's immune defense system by assisting in the production of antibodies and strengthening the white blood cells. Magnesium is helpful to many other functions which maintain normal cell development as well. Since a malignancy is caused by abnormal cell development, it's easy to see why magnesium is a necessary cancer preventive.

A diet which includes a lot of whole-grains, fruits, and vegetables should supply sufficient magnesium for healthy functioning. Authorities say that a dangerously low level of magnesium is rare, but can occur. For instance, a junk-food diet, chronic diarrhea, or a condition which interferes with proper assimilation of nutrients can set the stage for a magnesium deficiency.

SODIUM — Although sodium is rarely found in the makeup of a normal cell, the abnormal cancerous cell pumps sodium into itself. When a cell goes haywire and becomes malignant, it loses the calcium lining of its inner membranes, with magnesium and potassium also being lost. With the loss of calcium, the cell loses its normal defense capabilities. By absorbing sodium, the cancer cell places itself beyond the body's normal defenses.

The blood analyses of cancer patients commonly show that not only the malignancy, but the blood cells themselves are overloaded with sodium. A promising theory suggests that removing the sodium (desodification) from the cancer cells would open them once more to the body's immune system defenses. But what substance can modern medicine offer to selectively remove the sodium from the cancer cells? The answer to this problem may yet come from a killer who lives in the depths of the oceans.

CURRENTLY IN RESEARCH

SQUALENE — In the human body and in all animals, cancer rarely finds a home in the cartilage. But the cartilage of the shark's fin is even more resistant to cancer than human cartilage. In fact, as a species, sharks appear to have a built-in protection against cancer, and not just in their fin cartilage either. A study conducted under the auspices of the Smithsonian Institute in Washington, D.C. discovered only one malignant tumor in 25,000 sharks!

The shark secretes certain substances (taurine and isaethionic acid) in its liver which constantly recycle the high salt concentration of its environment back into the sea. In current medical practice, taurine is often prescribed for both migraine headaches and epilepsy. The shark's anticancer potential is incredibly high because it is in a constant process of desodification.

The shark has yet another method of suppressing cancer. Along with its ability to eliminate sodium, the shark produces an oily substance called squalene. Squalene is produced in large quantities in the shark's liver and is also found in smaller amounts in both cod liver oil and olive oil. Researchers believe that squalene restores the vital electrostatic balance which is lost when a cell turns cancerous. Once the balance is restored by the squalene, the body's defense system can identify, attack, and destroy the malignancy.

DHEA — Dehydroepiandrosterone (DHEA) levels in the blood apparently play a protective role against the development of cancer. It has been determined that when DHEA levels in the blood rise to a value of more than 3.3 mg, a cancer tumor goes into remission. Squalene appears to stimulate the body's own production of DHEA. It is known that approximately 60 percent of the population contains sufficient natural DHEA to be protected from cancer. Of the remaining 40 percent deficient in DHEA, it is theorized that more than half (22 percent) will die from cancer.

ALDEHYDES — The 'bitter almond' (Laetrile/Mandelonitrile) substances exert a gene-repairing effect on cancer cells. These substances include amygdalin, prunasin, cassavin, ficin, and the synthetic mandelonitril compounds. Benzaldehyde (one of the constituents of Laetrile) has been shown to have a very positive effect against cancer cells. The excellent experimental and clinical results achieved in Japan with benzaldehyde treatments were published by the National Cancer Institute as long ago as 1980.

Various forms of aldehyde cancer therapy have been practiced in Germany at the Paracelsus Hospital in Hannover for more than 15 years. A respected head nurse with many years of experience working with cancer patients at this prestigious institution says of the 'bitter almond' substances, "Among all forms of medical cancer treatment, including poisonous chemotherapy, this is still the best method."

RUBIDIUM & CESIUM — Both are nontoxic elements shown to be absorbed by a cancer cell. Once absorbed, they neutralize the harmful hydrogen ions present in the malignancy. Studies indicate that this treatment has a positive effect even when a cancer growth has attained considerable volume, but primarily assists the body's own immune system. These elements should therefore be administered early, before the defenses of the body have been damaged beyond repair.

UREA — Urea is a natural product of metabolized protein long used in medicine as a diuretic and in the diagnosis of kidney function. Urea therapy is considered inexpensive, harmless, and can be used for a long period. Results achieved at the Greek Cancer Clinic as far back as the early 1970s show that urea has strong antiviral properties and is therefore effective against viral-induced malignancies, such as liver cancer (hepatitis B) and oral tumors (herpes virus).

As a powerful diuretic, urea has been shown to detoxify the body by eliminating cancer degradation byproducts. The Greek studies published in 1974 list several case histories of cancer patients then in remission after receiving between 10 and 18 grams of urea daily.

ASSISTING INTERNAL DEFENSE MECHANISMS

STEROIDS — Certain lymphocytes (white blood cells) play a very important part in the defense systems of the body. Lymph cells function efficiently only when they are present in sufficient quantity. In order to possess the ability to inactivate a cancerous cell, lymphocytes require special steroids: *thymosterine* and *tumosterone*. In order to manufacture tumosterone, the body must first manufacture its precursor, thymosterine. And, in order to be able to manufacture the precursor thymosterine, the body requires Vitamin D2. Prednisone (but no other cortisone) is also a precursor of thymosterine. The steroids thymosterine and tumosterone are both activated by the thymus gland. A healthy thymus gland is absolutely vital to an efficiently functioning immune system.

It is believed that tumosterone moves directly into the nucleus of the malignant cell via the lymph and inactivates it. However, this can only occur if a lymphocyte with sufficient tumosterone has identified and attached itself to the cancer cell.

German researchers have broken down tumosterone chemically and have succeeded in identifying the final metabolite of this protective element as 7-beta-hydroxy-cholsterol. This means that tumosterone can now be produced in a laboratory.

SHEEP LICE — Sheep are extremely resistant to cancer, possibly because their wool-fat has been shown to be especially rich in tumosterone. An old-country cure for viral hepatitis has been practiced in Germany for centuries. It consists of eating sheep lice. This is just one more demonstration of a folk medicine strongly rooted in what we now know to be scientific fact.

THE IMMUNE SYSTEM — Although it is difficult to stimulate the functioning of the thymus gland directly, science can provide elements which assist the immune system. A continuing intake of bromelaine, abundant in pineapples, may be a useful aid to the immune system and is considered an excellent cancer-preventive as well. Gamma-globulin, zinc-aspartate, manganese-aspartate, and molybdenum (abundant in cauliflower), are considered helpful. It has been noted that zinc enhances the body's defenses against cancer and exerts a pronounced preventive effect. But, caution must be observed. Once a malignant tumor has become established, zinc may increase its rate of growth.

ANTITUBERCULOSIS VACCINE — Over twenty years ago, researchers discovered that an injection of the antituberculosis vaccine BCG (Calmette-Guerin bacillus) can activate two or three different defense procedures of the white blood corpuscles. Clinical trials showed that these internal defenses can be dramatically effective, even against advanced cancer. The use of the vaccine demands particular care, however. Unless the body's immune system is still functioning, the vaccine may shut it down entirely.

AT INCREASED RISK

Certain whole segments of the population are, on average,

at increased risk of developing some type of cancer within their lifetimes. For instance, employment in the rayon industry carries a higher cancer risk, just as miners risk developing black lung. Predicting who will and who will not develop a malignancy within any given group of persons is not an exact science because so many diverse factors influence health.

However, the following information deserves your close attention. You just might find that you or someone you love is in a high-risk group without even being aware of it. Identifying high-risk groups is the first step to assisting these groups in lowering their risk. This very vital information is unknown to most of the American public.

BLOOD TYPE A — Cancer cells develop a defense mechanism of their own by surrounding themselves with a camouflaging layer of mucus. This protective outer layer makes it difficult for the body's own defenses to recognize a malignant cell and they hesitate to attack it.

Those of us with blood type A are at particular risk of developing cancer at some time in our lives because cancerous cells have a marked resemblance to blood type A cells. The defense system present in blood group A is not efficient in idenifying cancer cells and is very slow to attack, thereby giving the cancer a better chance of developing.

German research has documented this problem. Blood type A represents 43 percent, less than half, of the German population. But a whopping 77 percent, more than three-quarters, of the cancer victims in that nation are blood type A. At the opposite end of the scale, the study showed that only 19 percent of Germany's cancer patients are blood type O, but blood type O carriers represents the highest percentage of the general population.

Clearly, blood type A (and AB) carriers should incorporate all the preventive measures known into their lifestyles as quickly as possible in order to reduce their risk of developing cancer.

THE HEREDITY FACTOR — A comforting statistic comes from A.G. Knudson, M.D., Ph.D., of the Fox Chase Cancer

Center (Philadelphia, Pennsylvania). This eminent scientist received the prestigious Scientific Achievement Award given by the American Cancer Society (Philadelphia Division) in 1984. Dr. Knudson says, "I'd estimate that about five percent of all cancers are purely heredity. These include certain childhood cancers and melanomas."

Dr. Knudson points out that some genetic defects have been identified as promoting the development of cancer in children. Cancer of the eye (retinoblastoma) is caused when a portion of the chromosome 13 is missing. A malformation of chromosome 8 causes Wilms' tumor. Malignant melanomas (cancerous moles) also appear to run in families. Dr. Knudson says it's important to realize that true "cancer families" are rare. He says, "Cancer families tend to inherit the same cancer or cancers, and to get the disease at an early age. There is one family in which 50 percent of the members develop the same kind of kidney cancer. That's very different from having an uncle who got lung cancer, a sister with breast cancer, and a mother with stomach cancer."

However, statistics do show that a woman whose mother or sister had breast cancer has a greater chance of developing breast cancer herself. And, says Dr. Knudson, some other cancers (colon, ovarian, nervous system) appear to have a genetic basis as well.

THE FAMILY AT RISK — It has long been noted that being born into a cancer-prone family appears to increase your risk of developing a malignancy at some time in your life. The American Institute for Cancer Research has begun an all-out offensive to discover why cancer seems to run in certain families.

The research has zeroed in on one particular oncogene called the Ha-*ras* gene. The term *oncogene* comes from the Greek word 'oncos' or tumor. Scientists theorize that oncogenes are present in all cells and believe their function is to regulate cell growth. Because cancer cells grow abnormally, learning what factor regulates normal cell growth is vitally important. Once the growth factor is identified, medical science may be able to develop a procedure to control the abnormal proliferation of cancer cells.

When viewed under a powerful electronic microscope, the Ha-*ras* gene reveals as many as 20 distinct different patterns. In an intensive study of this particular oncogene, both cancer patients and those in the control group were shown to carry four of the most common patterns. Of the sixteen less common Ha-*ras* patterns, 12 were found only in cancer patients.

This important research indicates that persons carrying the Ha-*ras* gene in one of the 12 suspect configurations are at higher risk of contracting cancer than their brothers and sisters who may not have inherited one of the problem patterns. Science may soon be able to perform a simple blood test to determine your genetic risk of developing a malignancy.

If you carry one of the Ha-*ras* genes commonly found in cancer patients, it does not automatically follow that you will absolutely develop cancer. Being forewarned is forearmed. What this means is that you should immediately take all possible steps to reduce your risk from outside factors. Although you cannot control your genetic inheritance, you can incorporate preventive measures into your lifestyle.

GEOPATHOGENIC ZONES

EARTH DISTURBANCES — What exactly are *geopathogenic* zones, probably a term new to most, if not all, of the American public? An examination of the word itself provides the explanation. *Geo* comes from the Greek and means 'the earth.' *Pathogenic* is defined as 'disease producing.' *What?* Are there then certain zones of the earth which foster the development of disease?

Unfortunately, the answer appears to be *yes.* As long ago as 1920, the world-renowned German surgeon and oncologist Dr. Sauerbruch advised his cancer patients not to return to their homes if they were in a geopathogenic zone. Research into the possibility of low-frequency electrical disturbances deep within the earth increasing the risk of cancer to those who live in the vicinity began seriously over twenty years ago by Dr. Ernst Hartmann of Eberbach, Germany.

In the beginning, Dr. Hartmann's theory was ridiculed by orthodox medicine, and is still rejected today by most cancer authorities. But science has now determined that even a very weak electromagnetic pulse (between 5 and 25 Hz) can produce cancer cells. These extremely low frequencies (ELF) are active in geopathogenic zones. The major cause of these harmful ELF is the underground water flowing beneath the surface of the earth. The veins and arteries carrying the life-sustaining water supplies of the world produce these dangerous low frequencies, which, in theory at least, foster the development of cancer in those living above them.

Further documentation comes from Dr. Nieper who reports the following as a result of his own research and continuing observation of the cancer victims he himself treats: "According to studies I initiated, at least 92 percent of all the cancer patients I examined have remained for long time periods — especially with respect to their sleeping place—in geopathogenic zones. In my opinion, it is essential that tumor patients, as well as patients suffering from multiple sclerosis, be apprised of this information and depart geopathogenic zones."

There are certain manufactured devices available which are purported to *shield* the user from the damaging effects of the geopathogenic zones. Shielding devices are not effective. However, there are some devices which can, but only in part, *neutralize* the harmful ELF. One such device, called the 'North-South Rectifier,' is manufactured by the Henry Weber Company, Switzerland and another comes from Eberbach in Germany. At this writing, no effective ELF neutralizing devices are available in the U.S.

ELECTRICAL FIELDS

FRIEND TURNED FOE — Substantiating even further the harmful effect of certain electrical fields is the fact that persons working in electric transformer stations have a higher incidence of leukemia. Research originating at the University of Colorado corroborates the suspicion that people living in the vicinity of powerful electric mains suffer a higher incidence of cancer than the general population.

Another factor which is not well-known in the U.S. is the damaging effects of alternating current. According to German studies, when electric blankets, heating pads, massage units, and the like are activated by alternating current, the ELF waves which radiate from these commonly used items inactivate the body's electrostatic filtering system, which normally keeps the urinary tract passages bacteria-free.

Experienced (and aware) oncologists have observed that from the end of August until the first cold frosty nights of the winter season, the body's immune defense capacity is reduced by up to 30 percent. There is a documented and dramatic increase in the rate of growth of any malignancy in the body during this time of year. Around August 28th, the planets in the solar system pass through a dense system of magnetic fields. Some researchers theorize that certain electromagnetic factors thus created contribute to a drop in the body's defense mechanisms. This effect continues until the planets move on in early January.

During the damp months of autumn and continuing until the first hard freeze of winter, any mother will tell you that her family is more subject to sore throats, coughs, colds, and flu. This phenomenon, long recognized, is at least partially due to the fact that the first freeze destroys airborne bacteria. However, now that science has determined that the immune system is not working at full capacity during the planetary configurations that occur during this period, researchers are taking a hard look at the possibility that electromagnetic pulses reaching the earth should figure into their calculations.

TEMPERATURE CONTROL — Another comfort of modern technology which can become a potential health hazard is the American practice of turning up the thermostat. Of particular importance to all of us, especially cancer patients, is the news that experiments have shown that the body's immune defense system becomes sluggish and its efficiency drops drastically at temperatures over approximately 64.5 degrees F. (18 degrees C.).

Perhaps my readiness to accept the effects of the planets on man stems from learning the proper phases of the moon for planting from my grandfather. Or perhaps it's the memory of my grandmother and her unwavering belief in the importance of assisting the body through natural dietary means to work at optimum efficiency. But can't help but observe that orthodox medicine seems determined to alter chemically (or cut out) rather than assist naturally by recommending the proper foods and supplements which are known to strengthen the body's immune defenses.

FLUORIDE IS POISON

Fluoride is another avoidable carcinogen. It is a documented fact that as little as one-tenth of an ounce of fluoride can cause death, yet all over the country, fluoride is routinely added to city water supplies as a dental caries (cavity) preventive. Statistics from the National Academy of Sciences indicate that U.S. industries pump over 100,000 tons of fluoride waste into the atmosphere every year and dump even more (an estimated 500,000 tons) into our waters. *Yes, fluoride is an industrial waste product* occurring in the production of aluminum. And, yes, it is this same industrial waste that is used to fluoridate our drinking water.

According to the 1983 *U.S. Pharmacopeia Volumes on Drug Information,* the following clinical signs of fluoride poisoning occur with alarming frequency among people ingesting tablets containing the amount of fluoride found in just 1 to 2 pints of fluoridated water: Black stool (tar-like), bloody vomiting, diarrhea, faintness, nausea, shallow breathing, stomach pain or cramps, tremors, unusual excitement, unusual increase in saliva, watery eyes, weakness, constipation, loss of appetite, bone involvement (aches and pains), skin rash, sores (mouth, lips), stiffness, weight loss, mottling of teeth (white, brown, or black discolorations).

FLUORIDE POISONINGS — A town in Kizilcaoren, Turkey has been dubbed *Das Dorf der jungen Greise,* "the village where people age before their time," by the German researchers studying this phenomenon. All the inhabitants of this area suffer from premature aging. Between the ages of 30 and 40, they develop the wrinkled skin typical of the normal

60 year old; young women give birth to dead babies after pregnancies of only 4 months duration; men of 30 are impotent; all suffer from a severe weakness of the musculoskeletal structure and walking is impossible without the support of a stick. Sick livestock slaughtered for food show diseased livers.

The slow and insidious poisoning of the villagers was uncovered by a dentist who noted the typical mottling (brown discoloration) of extreme fluoride poisoning on the teeth of all children over the age of 7 and complete discoloration of teeth in teenagers. Most adults in the village had just a few affected teeth remaining. When notified of this phenomenon, the medical staff at the University Clinic of Eskisehir, Turkey conducted an intensive investigation. Their report concluded that, on top of the reproductive difficulties and dental involvement pervading the population, "Every single inhabitant of Kizilcaoren suffers from a bone disease with symptoms including thickening of the ankles, stiffened joints, and abnormal growth of bone substance."

In neighboring Turkish villages where water is drawn from different sources, normal health prevails. But in Das Dorf der jungen Greise, water from the village well was found to contain an extremely high naturally-occurring fluoride concentration of 5.4 ppm (parts per million).

THE FLUORIDE/CANCER CONNECTION

THE IMMUNE SYSTEM — Scientists at the Seibersdorf Research Center in Austria have reported that as little as 1 ppm fluoride slows down the vitally important DNA repair enzyme activity of the immune system. It has long been noted that the higher incidence of cancer among older persons is directly related to the proven decline in the ability of the immune system to repair defective DNA components.

Numerous laboratory studies have shown that fluoridated water (at concentrations as low as 1 ppm) can cause serious genetic and chromosomal damage in plants, animals, and humans. Using bone marrow and testes cells, a U.S. geneticist has demonstrated that the degree of chromosomal damage increases proportionately as the fluoride content of the water increases. It is important to note that abnormal sperm cells which have been damaged by fluoride poisoning can lead to serious birth defects and certain metabolic disorders that can be passed on from generation to generation.

Using the same level of fluoride commonly put into U.S. water supplies, scientists at the Nippon Dental College in Japan have determined that this minute amount of fluoride is capable of transforming normal cells into cancer cells. At a meeting of the Japanese Association of Cancer Research in Osaka in 1982, the researchers reported, "Last year at this meeting we showed that sodium fluoride, which is being used for the prevention of dental caries, induces chromosomal aberrations and irregular synthesis of DNA. This year, we report our finding that a malignant transformation of cells is induced by sodium fluoride."

As incredible as it may seem, research sponsored by the American Cancer Institute as long ago as 1963 clearly showed that even very low levels of fluoride increased the incidence of melanotic tumors in experimental laboratory animals by a frightening 12 to 100 percent. Similar types of transformations of normal cells to potentially cancerous cells have been observed in humans.

Polish scientists working at the Pomeranian Medical Academy have published reports that as little as 0.6 ppm fluoride produces chromosomal damage in human white blood cells, the important defensive cells of the immune system.

SURPRISING FINDINGS

If some of this information comes as a surprise to you, we invite you to consider it carefully and incorporate whatever seems good and logical into your own lifestyle. Many of the preventive measures suggested are both inexpensive and simple. For instance, by merely adding carrot juice to your daily regimen, you will be providing your body with beta-carotene, an incredibly powerful cancer preventive.

I'll drink a toast to your health tomorrow morning at breakfast with my morning carrot juice! I recommend it highly.

Chapter XII
Healthy Living
A Summary of What's Good & What's Not

GOOD FOODS

LINSEED OIL — is at the very top of the list of good foods. This dietary fat is so vitally important to your health that we have devoted a great deal of space to explaining exactly what the essential fatty acids (linoleic and linolenic) do for you. We have explored the ways that linseed oil and cottage cheese, an excellent source of the sulphur-based proteins that activate the essential fatty acids, can dissolve tumors and restore even a terminal cancer victim to health. If you are skeptical of the wonders of crude linseed oil, please review Chapter 6 again.

We hate to remind you of the fact that the majority of U.S. brands of linseed oil generally don't measure up. There is however a product formulated from Europe that is from the first pressing of the seeds. You can trust that the essential fatty acids are present in rich abundance in virgin *C-Leinomed*™ (Linomed).

GARLIC — Garlic is mentioned several times within these pages as being a particularly healthy food. It has been used medically for centuries against congestion, circulatory problems, heart disease and more. As a powerful cancer preventive and therapeutic, garlic shows great promise. (See Chapter 4.)

I can't imagine anyone who doesn't enjoy this pungent herb, but if you just plain don't like garlic, you'll be interested in the newest garlic formulation to hit the market.*Garlimed*™ (garlic heals) is a new biologically active garlic preparation. Using the very latest technology, garlic cloves are harvested and processed straight from the garden to capture and preserve all the volatile oils and natural elements. The end result is a caplet containing all the vital health-promoting activity of this pungent herb. Studies comparing this method of processing with freshly harvested garlic show that the active constituents in both are the same. *Garlimed*™ — Ivan Robroff's original formula from Bulgaria—also contains hawthorn, hops, and rutin in an exclusive formulation which synergistically potentiates the scientifically documented healthful properties of the garlic itself.

Hawthorn promotes blood circulation through the coronary arteries and serves to maintain normal blood pressure. Garlic benefits the entire alimentary tract, especially where indigestion tends to occur. It helps normalize the blood pressure, particularly when fluctuation arises and acts on the cholesterol deposits in the blood vessels, thereby preventing the risk of arteriosclerosis. Hops helps to cleanse the blood, tone up the liver, stimulate a sluggish gallbladder and increase the flow of bile. It has a calming effect on the nervous system as it removes restlessness and promotes sleep. Rutin is a good source of bioflavonoids and helps the body utilize vitamin C. It strengthens fragile blood vessels and helps prevent their recurrent bleeding.

CARROTS — There's so much hard scientific evidence showing that the beta-carotene content of carrots alone qualifies this ancient root vegetable as an efficient cancer preventive and one which assists in the therapeutic treatment of fatty degeneration as well, that the point can hardly be argued. Carrots contain many important vitamins and minerals, making them exceptionally valuable nutritionally. As a raw addition to a salad, they offer a good quantity of sulphur-rich amino acids. A number of the vital alkaline elements are present in carrots in perfectly balanced proportions. These elements aid the body in many important functions, including the efficient assimilation of the essential fatty acids.

We remind you again that beta-carotene is fat-soluble and can only be used by the body in the presence of a fatty emulsion. The essential fatty acids the body requires are present in trace amounts in butter and cream, but, as we have discussed at length, a daily regimen which includes linseed oil and cottage cheese is a much healthier way to ingest these fats. (If you've forgotten the full story on carrots and beta-carotene, please see Chapters 4 and 11.)

FIBER FOODS — The average daily intake of fiber in the westernized and industralized nations is around 4 grams. In the so-called uncivilized countries, the daily fiber intake hovers around 30 grams, precisely the amount health experts recommend. Conditions of the digestive system and intestinal tract common to our society include constipation, a national problem continuing to grow by astronomical proportions. Other disorders include cancer of the colon, diverticulosis and diverticulitis, diseases of the large intestine and rectum, and hemorrhoids. These conditions are uncommon in areas where fiber intake is high.

Two generations ago, our daily diet included a lot of what grandmother called 'roughage.' Grandmother served brown rice and cereal grains that were unmilled and unrefined, and she usually baked her own bread. She put a lot of raw vegetables fresh from the garden on the table, or cooked them with the skins on to 'save vitamins.' We enjoyed our fruits sun-warmed and ate them whole, ingesting a lot of healthy fiber in the bargain.

Today, fruits turn up as a jumble of bits and pieces in a can labeled 'fruit cocktail.' The fiber that was in the skin has been discarded. orange juice is now filtered and 'concentrated,' with all the sweet pulp removed. The pulp and white membrane that separates the sections, rich in fiber, has been thrown away. Today, we have to eat 16 slices of commercially baked white bread (made with hydrogenated oils, another warning sign) in order to consume the 30 grams of fiber contained in just 4 slices of whole-grain bread. Are you beginning to track the clues to the problem here?

Another important factor in favor of fiber is that it contains no calories, meaning that it can't go to your waist (or hips). Fiber passes through the body virtually unchanged. It supplies bulk needed by the intestines to remove body wastes with such haste that they don't have time to putrify and cause irreparable harm. (See Chapter 3 for a fast review of how fiber works as a cancer preventive.) However, a high fiber diet acts to leach some important minerals from the system and quickly excretes them. When adding fiber to your diet, make sure your diet also contains foods rich in calcium (dairy products, eggs, beans, cauliflower), magnesium (whole grains, vegetables, fruits), and zinc (milk, liver, shellfish, herring, wheat bran). (Note: As a powerhouse containing *all* essential nutrients, bee pollen is a good natural source of these three minerals.)

The recommendations are clear, but if your dietary habits are too firmly entrenched to make the necessary changes, a product called *Fibermed-7*™ may be your answer. Along with healthy natural herbal fiber, this important supplement contains a measure of calcium, magnesium, and zinc, precisely the minerals the body especially needs when additional fiber is added to the diet. With apple fiber, oat fiber, alfalfa, carob, apple pectin, arrow root, cellulose, dandelion root, marshmallow root, oat straw, slippery elm, and Chinese cinnamon, plus the vital minerals listed above, the ingredients in this product might have been selected by Mother Nature herself. In convenient caplet form, *Fibermed 7*™ has the rather pleasant taste of nature in the raw, and may be chewed for faster assimilation, if desired. This is the easy way to supplement your diet with healthy fiber.

Note: Although fiber itself has no caloric value, fiber-rich foods contain varying amounts of calories. For those on a weight-loss regimen, taking a fiber supplement might be the wiser course. For example, eating 4 slices of delicious whole-grain bread will easily supply the day's optimum amount of fiber, but there are times when eating this amount of bread will add some unwanted and unnecessary calories to the menu.

RAW FOODS — After the traditional Thanksgiving feast, a big Sunday dinner, or other heavy meal, we usually push back from the table, yawn, and feel so tired we're impelled to take a snooze. We put that tired feeling down to overeating, and that's part of it, but there's a further explanation. When we feed on cooked (dead) food, the body fights back. The stomach and intestinal tract reacts to the mass of cooked foods by rushing white blood cells to the scene and with swelling or bloating. The temperature in the localized area rises and develops a 'fever.' In case you didn't recognize this reaction, it is the same reaction the body exhibits in the presence of an infection *and* around a tumor.

Cooking destroys all the living digestive enzymes in food. The body is forced to secrete an extra supply of digestive enzymes in order to process the dead mass. Late-breaking research coming out of Europe tells us that the body reacts in the same way when just part of the meal is eaten cooked and part of the meal is eaten raw — *if* the cooked food is ingested first. However, if we first eat some raw foods before consuming the cooked portion of the meal, the reaction does not occur.

A very few foods are not good for us in their raw state. Raw potatoes are just not tasty, even though their nutritional value is high. Raw beans contain a protein-like substance *(phaseolin)* which can cause indigestion. Raw egg whites contain another protein-like element *(avidin)* which inhibits the absorption of important B vitamins. Avidin is destroyed in cooking. (If you enjoy a protein shake made in your blender, don't use raw eggs as part of the ingredients.)

But it's delightful to begin a meal with a big salad of leafy greens and raw vegetables. Make sure your salad contains shredded carrots, garlic, green (or red) bell peppers, hot peppers (if you like them), radishes, and onions along with dark green leafy 'lettuces.' Spinach is one of the best. Dress your salad with one of the linseed oil and cottage cheese based salad dressing recipes given in Chapter 7 and give your long-suffering stomach a rest!

BEE POLLEN — For a healthy helping of live enzymes, there's no better source than a high quality bee pollen. The golden granules of this nutritional sunshine from the beehive, when correctly handled, are richly enzyme active and a superior source of all the nutrients (amino acids, vitamins, minerals, essential fatty acids, hormones, carbohydrates, trace elements) required by the life processes. As a cancer fighter, bee pollen has been shown in scientifically controlled double-blind studies to inhibit the development of tumors. Also, cancer victims undergoing radiation therapy found the debilitating side-effects of this form of treatment were reduced and easier to bear when they were given bee pollen.

Our vote for the best bee pollen goes to a relative newcomer to the scene. *Desert Gold Crown*™ (granules) and *Bee Pollemed Gold*™ (capsule formula) from Biowell is harvested in areas free of environmental contamination, is cold processed to protect enzymatic activity, is a blended multisource product, and is packaged in pharmaceutical quality bottles to insure all properties remain active and potent. Both Montana Pollen & Herb's *Big Sky* and C C Pollen Company's *High Desert*® are also good choices. (See Chapter 8.)

SUSPECT FOODS

SUGAR — When we eat food (carbohydrates), it is true that the body sorts out all the elements and eventually breaks down the constituents into simple sugars (glucose and fructose). *Glucose* is the major sugar present in blood and body tissues. This is an essential sugar in that all cells, especially brain cells, depend on glucose. But there is no RDA (Recommended Daily Allowance) for any kind of sugar, including glucose. We are not required to eat a measure of glucose every day. The specialized enzymes of the digestive tract are equipped to convert carbohydrates into the basic glucose the body needs. Glucose is released slowly into the bloodstream during the metabolic process, along with other needed nutrients.

One of the most common misconceptions today, fostered by some excellent advertising, is that white sugar (which is not glucose, but *sucrose*) provides quick energy and is a good food. The catch is that sugar is not absorbed and metabolized in the body in the same efficient way as complex carbohydrates are. When we eat sugar, it is rapidly absorbed and passed on to the liver where it is converted into triglycerides. The triglycerides are released into the bloodstream and end up being stored as fat deposits in the veins and tissues. Do we have to remind you that high cholesterol and triglyceride levels are implicated in the development of cancer, heart disease, and many other life-threatening conditions?

An intake of sugar also triggers the release of insulin by the pancreas. The insulin metabolizes the sugar rapidly in order to maintain normal blood-sugar levels. But the sugar is digested and assimilated so quickly that a lot of excess insulin (with a much longer half-life than sugar) continues racing around the bloodstream and is left with nothing to process. This is the big reason why sugar picks you up fast, but lets you down even faster. Sugar is not a source of sustained energy at all. The ingestion of large amounts of sugar over a long period of time places tremendous stress on the pancreas. Diabetes results when the pancreas is exhausted and loses its ability to synthesize insulin. Diabetes (and related side effects) ranks third (after heart disease and cancer) as a cause of death in America.

CHEMICAL FOOD ADDITIVES — You're having a few people in for the evening. In your best party snack bowls, you serve your guests some citric acid mixed with propylene glycol, a variety of glycerides, some butylated hydroxyanisole, butylated hydroxytoluene, propyl gallate, chemically-altered fats, and an excessive amount of sodium, plus, of course, a measure of dye and artifical flavoring. All this yucky stuff is part of the ingredients you usually find in a bag of corn chips. Still hungry?

As of 1983, the FDA had approved the use of more than 3,000 food additives. The number of additives listed as GRAS (Generally Regarded As Safe at a specified level) in 1983 totaled over 1,000. Today, some authorities estimate that as many as 7,000 chemicals appear in our foods.

The food industry spends over *20 billion dollars* every year on the chemical additives they put in our food. An educated guess is that each of us consumes over five pounds of chemical preservatives, stabilizers, dyes, artificial flavorings, and other additives each year without really thinking much about it.

These chemicals serve a variety of purposes. They act as bleaching agents, extenders, clarifiers, emulsifiers, softeners, thickeners, hydrogenators, curing agents, buffers, deodorizers, sprout inhibitors, fungicides, sweeteners, conditioners, antioxidants, fortifiers, drying agents, alkalizers, defoamers, firming agents, stabilizers, and preservatives.

We have to depend on the FDA to test and approve (or disallow) food additives. New substances are tested on lab animals and those that prove deadly within 24 hours to two weeks of ingestion are evaluated further. Another test is to determine what quantity of a substance must be ingested to kill half the animals during the experimental period. This is the test used to determine 'safe' levels of ingestion for humans.

Unfortunately, there is no established testing procedure to discover the effects of ingesting a *combination* of chemicals, something we do every day. Interestingly enough, the FDA itself has shown that consuming just *one-tenth* of the fatal amount (presumably a 'safe' level) of two different chemicals at the same time can result in death. It's impossible for science to establish 'safe' levels of ingestion of a potentially dangerous substance without knowing exactly what substances we might consume along with it.

Most food additives are nutritionally valueless. Additives are used mainly to make inferior foods cosmetically attractive, to make them 'convenient' to prepare, and to extend shelf life. *We really do know there's a better way to eat,* but the food industry mounts massive advertising campaigns to convince us otherwise. And we let ourselves be persuaded. Here's a quick review of some of the common food additives we eat every day:

BHA & BHT — Butylated hydroxyanisole (BHA) and butylated hydroxytoluene (BHT) are popular antioxidants which are used to prevent foods (in which the natural antioxidants have been refined out) from going rancid on the shelves over a long period. These petroleum-based chemicals have been banned in Great Britain and many other countries of the world, but the powerful food processors in the U.S. equate long shelf life with corporate profits. It's my guess that BHA and BHT will be with us for a long time. You'll find BHA and BHT in cereals, candy, gelatin, shortening, ice cream, dairy foods, processed meats, peanut butter, margarine, chewing gum, vegetable oils, dried fruits, meats, fish, salad dressings, most popular snack foods, and much more.

Lead — Canned meats and milk may become contaminated with lead (from the seal on the can), but we also take in lead unwittingly from toothpaste, aluminum foil, car exhausts, factory wastes, and other canned foods.

MSG — Monosodium glutamate has been around a long time. In 1968, researchers at Washington University determined that excessive intake damaged brain cells in lab animals. As a result of these findings, baby food manufacturers discontinued use of MSG. Just one-quarter teaspoon of MSG can upset the digestive processes and produces an allergic reaction in many infants.

Nitrates — In combination with nitrosamines, nitrates pose an unnecessary cancer risk. The American Cancer Society has recommended we sharply reduce our consumption of cured and processed meats (ham, bacon, sausage, hot dogs, cold cuts) because of their content of nitrates and nitrites. (For more, see Chapter 4.)

'ENRICHED' BREADS — Are you fooled by the word 'enriched' on that spongy supermarket bread? Here's the inside story:

Monostearates — Monostearates are classified as 'emulsifiers.' An emulsifier causes flour to absorb up to six times its own weight in water. In humans, it acts on tissues and cells and increases their absorption capacity. This means we are likely to absorb toxins and poisons at an accelerated rate. Laboratory animals fed monostearates developed diarrhea and ulcerations, bled internally all along the genito-urinary tract, and died within weeks. Studies show that monostearates cause cancer in rats.

Propionates — Propionates are used to slow down the growth of molds, making the bread appear fresh longer. Propionates (also a prime ingredient in ointments and powders for treating athlete's foot) are steam-processed from ethylene and carbon monoxide and interfere with the body's ability to assimilate calcium.

Inorganic Calcium — The synthetic form of calcium used to 'enrich' breads can't be assimilated by the body anyway.

Ammonium Chloride — Powdered soaps and detergents, antifreeze, and many breads contain this chemical. In bread making, it is used to ferment dough.

Potassium Bromate — Many home permanents contain potassium bromate; the label carries a warning not to drink it. In bread making, potassium bromate holds in air bubbles while the loaf is baking, providing the spongy texture.

Inorganic Iron — The form of iron (ferrum radactum) used to enrich most breads can't be assimilated or used by the body.

Chemically-Altered Fats — Most breads are made with hydrogenated or partially hydrogenated fats. (See Chapter 5.)

Refined Flour — With all its healthy fiber stripped away, and most vitamins and minerals eliminated in the refining process, the nutrient value of refined flour breads is questionable. Do we need to remind you that The American Cancer Society says fiber is an important part of the anticancer diet? A diet deficient in fiber promotes obesity. We overeat refined low-nutrient foods because the body tries desperately to secure the nutrients it needs to function. A high fiber diet also prevents constipation and related problems, such as hemorrhoids.

THE HAZARDS OF EATING OUT — Walk into any restaurant, tell the maitre d' (or manager) you're allergic to *sulfites,* ask if sulfites are in the foods they serve, and you'll probably be rewarded with a blank stare. Nowdays, most restauranteurs can tell you they don't cook with MSG, and many will say they don't use sulfites on their salad greens or fresh vegetables, but most are unaware of the sulfites in commercially processed foods.

Sulfites — Although asthmatics who ingest sulfites are at greater risk than most of us, about 25 percent of the complaints received by the FDA regarding sulfites come from persons who don't have a history of asthma. Symptoms of sulfite sensitivity include: severe respiratory distress, vomiting, nausea, diarrhea, abdominal pain and cramps, hives, unconsciousness and death. At least 20 deaths associated with sulfite consumption had been reported to the FDA by 1985.

In one or the other of its many disguises, sulfites function as preservatives and/or antioxidants. Some are used as bleaching agents for food starches, some are used in the manufacturing of cellophane, and some are used as sterilizing agents. Salad fixings are dipped or dusted with sulfites to preserve their fresh look and appetizing color.

Sulfites include a variety of sulfur-based additives (sulfur dioxide, sodium sulfite, sodium and potassium bisulfite, sodium and potassium metabisulfite). You'll find sulfites in baked goods, chip dips, dried fish, canned or dried fruits, juices, gelatin, potato products, salad dressings, relishes, sauces, gravies, sauerkraut, cole slaw, shellfish (fresh, frozen, canned), dried and canned soups, vegetables (frozen, dried, canned), vinegars, wine, beer, and cider.

It's hard to understand just how sulfites have assumed such importance. People have been baking for centuries without sulfites. People have been drying fish, vegetables, fruits, and even meats for centuries without sulfites. People have been eating shellfish for centuries without sulfites. People have been making wine, beer, and cider for centuries without adding sulfites. When I was a child, I remember my grandmother making sauerkraut (and many other cabbage dishes) without sulfites. The only reason sulfites are added to our foods today is to improve the look of inferior foods and extend the shelf life.

HERE'S HOW TO FIGHT BACK

Money talks. If enough of us simply stop buying over-processed foods over-laden with chemical additives (or with their original nutrients chemically altered into alien elements that the body doesn't recognize and can't metabolize), the food processors will get the message. Food processors are in business to make money. Health-food stores are picking up customers by leaps and bounds as more and more people become aware of the dangers of chemically-laced foods.

Organically-Grown — The producers of organically grown produce (and meats) are now being actively sought out by those 'in the know' who want to avoid the profusion of harmful chemicals creeping into the food chain courtesy of giant agribiz executives. These giant producers are more interested in bringing food animals to market size in a hurry, and in growing ever-larger food crops by taking advantage of chemical technology, than they are in producing nutritious food.

Yes, you do pay more for foods certified as being organically produced, and that's a large stumbling block for many of us. But, it might very well be a question of 'pay now' or 'pay later' in the form of increased medical bills.

As biochemists and medical science learn more about the workings of human cells and genetics, the far-reaching implications of this constant consumption of chemicals becomes truly alarming. It is frighteningly obvious that we don't know enough about the *cumulative* effects of food additives, and it may take many years (possibly generations) before the effects are fully manifested.

And this is exactly the way cancer (and other degenerative diseases) work. One single cell gone wrong can be the start. Over time (sometimes as long as 10 or 20 years), a slow growing malignancy develops until the symptoms finally become noticeable.

We can't blame all our health problems on the food industry. The law of supply and demand comes into play. If processed foods weren't selling (and we spend billions of dollars on them every year), the industry would immediately replace them with food items more to our liking. If the newest convenience food doesn't grab its share of our food dollars, it's gone. Market researchers know exactly what the consumer buys.

SHOPPING IN THE ENEMY CAMP — If you're armed with enough knowledge (and we're trying), you can safely shop for most of your food needs in a supermarket. But what you *must* do is learn to read labels.

Sugar — A reminder that sugar is in just about everything. Sugar contributes to diabetes and hypo/hyperglycemia. It provides nothing but empty calories that the body doesn't need or want. *You* may have trained your body to crave processed sweets, but it knows better. Try honey instead. *Note:* Honey is a natural sweet, but is even more strongly implicated in the development of dental decay than sugar. Why? Because of its viscosity, it clings to the teeth longer than sugar. (You should be brushing after every meal anyway.)

Cola Drinks — If you drop a human tooth into a cola, it begins to dissolve in just 48 hours.

Soft Drink Powders — These popular products are dyed chemicals with artificial flavors. The 'sugarless' varieties usually contain NutraSweet® . (See 'NutraSweet® ' this chapter.)

Juices — I can't imagine why natural sweets have to be sugared. It's hard to find any juice (fruit or vegetable) in the supermarket that doesn't contain added sugar in some form, but it can be done. Read the label before you bring it home.

Fresh Produce — You're on safer ground here. The fresh produce in the supermarket hasn't been organically grown and may be lower in nutrients than products grown nature's way, but at least it isn't refined. Ask the produce manager if they use sulfites, and remember to watch out for irradiated foods. (See 'Nuked Foods' this chapter.) vegetables and fruits are rich in vitamins, mineral, nutrients, and fiber the mainstay of a healthy diet.

Whole-Grain Products — When buying breads (crackers, snacks) read the label carefully. Don't buy products made with refined flours or hydrogenated/partially hydrogenated oils. Whole wheat bread isn't necessarily made with the *whole* grain. Check the label to see if the bran (outer covering) and germ are in there.

Cereals — There are many cereal boxes to read, but do it. You'll really be surprised to find how few brands are made *with* the whole grain and *without* added sugar.

Meat, Fish, Poultry — Never buy any processed meats. Forget about frozen fish with a 'crispy' coating, but do enjoy fresh or frozen fillets (baked or poached). Skin poultry to reduce saturated fat consumption.

Yes, You Can — You can avoid eating all those chemicals. Read labels, be prepared to do a little extra work in the kitchen, and shop wisely.

NUTRASWEET® — This is just one more artificial chemical substance that far too many of us have embraced with open arms. We thought you ought to know that this chemical sweetener isn't as good as its advertising. G.D. Searle & Co. has succeeded in popularizing NutraSweet® through a systematic multi-million dollar advertising campaign. It is now widely used in diet drinks, chewing gum, puddings, and other products. The big attraction of NutraSweet® appears to be because it is perceived to be an 'easy way' to lose weight while still enjoying the sweet taste that many dieters crave.

The manufacturer claims this a popular low-calorie sweetener is as natural as bananas with milk. One of the major ingredients of NutraSweet® is *phenylalanine,* an amino acid. Dr. Richard J. Wurtman of the Massachusetts Institute of Technology believes that consuming large amounts of phenylalanine-laced NutraSweet® raises the levels of the chemical phenylalanine in the brain, thus interfering with the body's production of important neurotransmitters that protect against seizures. Anything that upsets the delicate chemical balance of the brain has to qualify as *bad,* to my way of thinking.

Dr. Wurtman, publishing in the well respected British journal *Lancet,* cites cases of individuals suffering their first epileptic seizures after drinking large quantities of beverages sweetened with NutraSweet®. On top of seizures, common complaints include mood changes, severe headaches, nausea, hallucinations, abnormal breathing, and night twitching. One unfortunate victim suffered a seizure while sleeping, and many NutraSweet® fans have had to be hospitalized.

The most recent development in the NutraSweet® controversy concerns The Community Nutrition Institute, a consumer group. On behalf of all of us, this group is petitioning the Food & Drug Administration asking for an immediate ban on NutraSweet®. An attorney for CNI, who has spent 15 years questioning the safety of this chemical sweetener, says conclusively: "The FDA no longer knows whether this product is safe."

This latest challenge to NutraSweet® is backed up by some hard clinical evidence. Researchers at the Massachusetts Institute of Technology in Cambridge have reported that more than 80 people suffered brain seizures after eating or drinking products containing aspartame (NutraSweet®). The study is an attempt to determine what changes in the brain chemistry are triggered by ingesting NutraSweet®. These are not isolated occurrences either. Across the country, more and more individuals are discovering that they experience disturbing symptoms ranging from mild to severe while taking NutraSweet® or NutraSweet® sweetened commercial products.

The CNI petition cites this new research and states: "The existence of these 80 cases meets the FDA's own definition of an imminent hazard to the public health, which requires the FDA to expeditiously remove a product from the market." The Institute maintains there is evidence that *NutraSweet® causes brain damage, cancer, and harm to fetuses.*

A spokesman for the FDA has said that the agency's view of NutraSweet® has not changed since the chemical sweetener was approved for use in dry foods in 1981 and in carbonated beverages in 1983. In the meantime, the FDA continues to evaluate consumer complaints, which are escalating.

Dr. Gerald Gaull, Vice President of Nutrition & Medical Affairs for NutraSweet®, says: "We have no new scientific evidence that in any way suggests that our product is anything but completely safe." We can only conclude that Dr. Gaull has declined to review the recent MIT research showing that brain seizures have occurred in 80 individuals after the ingestion of NutraSweet®.

The Community Nutrition Institute petition notes that the FDA has recently solicited proposals for an in-depth study into the effects on the brain of such substances as aspartame. In the legal arguments accompanying the petition, attorneys for CNI state emphatically: "The FDA is unable to say at this time that 'no harm' is being caused by aspartame (NutraSweet®). At best, the FDA is able to say only that it is likely that the harm being alleged against aspartame is coming from new areas of science that the agency failed to examine during the approval process."

It has been shown that aspartame can break down into methyl alcohol (a toxic poison) when stored at high temperatures. With the evidence against NutraSweet® continuing to build, wouldn't it be better to eliminate this harmful artificial chemical sweetener from your diet immediately? As a relative newcomer to the food chain, NutraSweet® hasn't been around long enough to judge its cumulative effects in the body. And, even though the symptoms of NutraSweet® poisoning (usually) disappear within a few weeks of discontinuing use, why risk your good health when Mother Nature's sweet fruits are available in abundance everywhere?

'NUKED' FOODS — *What* — In early 1986, the Federal Government approved the use of radiation to kill insects on fruits and vegetables. During this process, the food is chemically changed, but Radiation Technology, Inc. (Rockaway, New Jersey) tells us that the change in nutrient value is 'nominal.'

When — Irradiating of some pork products began a while back when the FDA approved a special petition from a pork packer. Because approval was sought by petition from an outside company, the FDA was not bound to publish proposed regulations and solicit consumer reaction. Critics had 30 days to protest, but not enough of us knew about it. You may have been eating irradiated pork since mid-1985 without knowing it.

Where — By the time you read this, even more irradiated products will be in supermarkets all over the country. By law, for the next two years, all foods thus treated must carry the words 'treated by radiation' (or 'irradiation') and must display the international symbol of this treatment.

The symbol is a broken circle with a small ball and two leaves in the middle. Watch for it. The only way you'll be able to tell if you are purchasing (and eating) radiated food is to spot the symbol. You can't see a difference and you can't taste a difference. The chemical disarrangment of the atoms and electrons in foods thus treated are both invisible and tasteless.

Irradiation Symbol

Certain fruits are targeted for processing with radiation. Peaches, strawberries, melons, nectarines, and papayas — the harvest of summer are the most likely candidates. We are told that 'nuked' fruits may be more expensive because the process is new. We are supposed to be thankful because they will last longer than their natural untreated cousins.

Why — Radiation does, we are assured, extend the shelf life of the foods thus treated. This undoubtedly will benefit the food industry, but what does it mean to the consumer? Unfortunately, no one knows. The process is too new for anyone to know exactly what the long term effects of eating 'nuked' foods might be.

WHY CONSUMER CONCERN IS JUSIIFIED — Some scientists and many health authorities say this process raises more questions than can be answered at the present time. We just don't know exactly what the chemical changes radiation causes in foods will do in the body. It has been determined that most of the x-rays used to bombard the food in this process do pass straight through without changing the intrinsic structure of the food itself. So far, so good. It's the rays that remain behind in the food that are causing concern.

URPs — True, these electrons do kill insects, destroy the bacteria that cause spoilage, and inhibit the ripening process to insure a longer shelf life. But they destroy certain natural bonds in the food and also bind with the natural elements to

223

create entirely new chemical substances that Mother Nature never heard of. These newly created chemicals which are found to occur in radiation treated foods have been dubbed URPs (*unique radiolytic products*). Virtually nothing is known about them or their possible effects on health.

Concerned consumer groups like the Public Citizen Health Research Group (Washington, D.C.) point out that the only way to determine if the URPs are toxic or worse, cancer-causing, is by feeding these substances to laboratory animals in the usual long-term controlled testing procedures. To date, studies sponsored by the U.S. Department of Agriculture with foods exposed to high levels of radiation found some serious dangers to health, including damage to the testes (and testicular tumors), a decease in the number of offspring, and lowered survival rates.

Although studies have not shown that irradiated foods are safe, and current FDA policy requires extensive testing of food chemicals (which has not been done with radiated food), for some reason the Food & Drug Administration appears to be ignoring its own safety regulations in this case. The Health Research Group says that the FDA's decision to allow irradiation of foods is based on *estimates* of the amount of URPs which may be produced during processing, and not on actual scientific evidence. We are back to square one. No one really knows what effects radiated foods can or will have in the body.

Changes in Nutrient Values — Early studies show that radiation can affect the vital essential fatty acids and amino acids in natural foods. In addition, some destruction of vitamins A, B, C, and E will occur. But the FDA says that radiation at the relatively low levels allowed are not a cause for consumer fears. A spokesman for the agency says that the FDA will "look into these concerns further before allowing higher levels."

Critics of the process point out that radiation may destroy the bacteria in foods which cause an unpleasant smell or other obvious signs of spoilage without completely destroying the harmful organisms themselves. This means that we just might end up buying foods that look and smell fresh, but which harbor harmful bacteria.

Consumer groups say that the amount of radioactive materials that will go in and out of just one food irradiation plant (three are projected) every five years will be five times the volume of low-level nuclear wastes produced in the U.S. by *all* sources in 1981, the latest year for which figures are available. Disposing of nuclear power waste is already a serious problem, with many states banning transport across their state boundaries. And we still haven't touched on the dangers to workers, the environment, and the local community in the event of an accident.

Incidentally, the Energy Department is offering waste from nuclear weapons production for the irradiation of foods. That's one way to dispose of 'hot' waste for a profit. First they dump aluminum byproduct wastes (fluoride) in our drinking water (See FLUORIDE this chapter), and now they're using nuclear waste to 'nuke' our foods.

What Can We Do To Protect Ourselves? — Soon the federal government will begin a campaign aimed at persuading America of the 'benefits' and 'safety' of irradiated foods. Don't be fooled. Write to state, local, and U.S. officials of your legitimate concerns. The ultimate protest is simply to refuse to purchase radiated foods. Alert your friends and neighbors to the facts and talk to supermarket owners. If an informed public boycotts 'nuked' foods en masse, the manufacturers and food sellers watching their profit margins drop will get the message in a hurry.

COFFEE & TEA — Along with that caffeine boost you think you need, you are ingesting other substances completely alien to the blood (theobromine, theine, tannin). These toxic elements enter the bloodstream and are carried to the brain, heart, pancreas, spleen, and other organs and glands. The liver and kidneys try valiantly to cleanse and detoxify the contaminated blood and often end up overtired, overworked, and exhausted by their efforts.

If you usually consume a lot of coffee and/or tea, but doubt they are addictive, try eliminating them from your diet abruptly. You'll probably experience withdrawal symptoms ranging from violent headaches to nausea to the shakes. If your health is important to you, it's worth going through the withdrawal period. Science confirms that simply eliminating coffee, and tea (plus cocoa and soda drinks) from the diet can result in a healthy reduction of high blood pressure, reduces the load on the heart, and reopens the arteries supplying the brain.

ANIMAL FATS — For the first time since 1978, the American Heart Association has issued an update on what they call the 'Healthy Heart Dietary Guidelines.' According to Heart Association data, released at a news conference in Washington, D.C. on August 26, 1986, over half a million Americans will die this year of heart disease. They estimate that upwards of 63 million of us have some form of heart dysfunction and serious blood vessel involvement right now.

The American Heart Association has declared all-out war on the 54 billion dollar per year fast food industry by targeting hamburgers as the number one source of saturated fats in the American diet. According to Association statistics, the hamburger accounts for 20 percent of the saturated fat intake on American menus. The 'Healthy Heart' guidelines call for saturated fats to be limited to a scant 10 percent of our daily calorie count, but current consumption totals between 15 and 20 percent and is viewed as a serious threat to health.

Note: The Heart Association dietary guidelines also say that we should reduce sodium consumption to 2½ grams (one teaspoon) per day. We are also advised to eat more fresh vegetables and fruits, more greens, lean meats and fish, and take only low-fat dairy products. The American Cancer Society is in full agreement with the American Heart Association. Please see Chapter 4 for a complete review of the ACS guidelines.

Without exception, medical authorities everywhere agree that we simply must reduce our consumption of saturated animal fats. If you're a fast-food fanatic and resist giving up your greasy burgers, try these figures on for size. The *Center for Science in the Public Interest* (Washington, D.C.) recently tested and rated the almighty all-American hamburgers produced by some of the more popular burger palaces across the country for saturated fat content. Here's what they found out:

SATURATED FAT CONTENT
IN FAST-FOOD HAMBURGERS

- *Carl's Jr.* — The Famous Star Burger
  — 23.6 percent fat
- *Jack in the Box* — The Jumbo Jack
  — 23.4 percent fat
- *Denny's* — regular hamburger
  — 22.3 percent fat
- *Hardee's* — regular hamburger
  — 21.7 percent fat
- *Roy Rogers* — regular hamburger
  — 21.3 percent fat
- *McDonald's* — Quarter Pounder
  — 20.2 percent fat
- *Burger King* — Whopper
  — 20.1 percent fat
- *Wendy's* — regular hamburger
  — 20.6 percent fat
- *D'Lites* — The D'Lite
  — 17.1 percent fat

It appears that we like our hamburgers greasy and full of fat. While we're still on the subject of burgers, a homemade burger (broiled) made with regular ground beef (which is 70 to 75 percent fat before cooking) ends up containing around 19.8 percent fat.

You'll be a little better off if you opt for fast roast beef, but keep in mind you'll still be consuming saturated animal fat. *Arby's* regular roast beef sandwich registered a relatively low 13 percent fat, but is made with processed beef consisting of chunks of untrimmed sirloin and round processed with water, salt, and food-grade phosphates. We are misled into believing we're getting 'roast beef' like mother used to make because the firm then packs the blend into the shape of a roast. *Roy Rogers* roast beef *is* roast beef (top round with the fat trimmed) and came in at only 1.4 percent fat.

Note: After pointing an accusing finger at many of the fast-food chains above, we should add a word of praise here for

Denny's. This chain has prepared a series of four brochures about their various food offerings which are available at the cash register, free for the taking.

Here's a quick booklet review: *Dine to your Heart's Content* lists Denny's menu items which are said to follow the American Heart Association guidelines and shows the cholesterol content of each. *Salt Away* helps consumers on low sodium diets choose low-salt foods and shows the content of sodium in many selections. This booklet also informs us that a salt-substitute is available on request. *For Sensitive People* targets foods prepared with MSG (monosodium glutamate), sulfites, and lactose — common food additives that cause an allergic reaction in many. *Waist Not, Want Not* offers a quick review of menu items with 550 calories or less for weight-watchers. It also provides some low-calorie substitution suggestions, such as using lemon and vinegar in place of a high-calorie salad dressing, and touts a low calorie syrup, which is available on request. Three cheers for Denny's for making this important nutritional information readily available to their patrons.

COWS' MILK — As long as we're attacking all the sacred cows that have become so firmly entrenched in our culture, we might as well say a word here about the fat content of the cows' milk we put on the family table as well. We have long been taught that cows' milk is the perfect food, and so it is — for calves. We don't take it directly from the cow herself, of course.

Cows' milk usually comes to us pasteurized, homogenized and frosty cold, very appetizing indeed, especially when served in clear crystal. We urge our children: 'Drink your milk, dear. It makes strong bones and teeth.' However, I remind you that man is the only creature in the world who continues *unnecessarily* to drink milk after being weaned. If you question the truth of that statement, you should know that the enzymes the human body requires to digest milk gradually disappear and are no longer available to the body after age three.

The elements present in both mothers' milk and cows' milk varies according to the diet taken by the donor. The fatty acid content of cows' milk totals about 3.5 percent, with only a very small percentage of the total fat content in the form of the essentials (linoleic and linolenic). But the inner construction of the cow's four stomachs results in a heavy secretion of bacteria which saturates and destroys the value of the essential fatty acids. (See *Butter* Chapter 5.)

The dairy industry could provide the cow with special feed, shown in tests to boost the percentage of usuable essential fats present in the milk, but this especially processed feed is very expensive. Another drawback is that the milk from cows fed this type of feed tastes unpleasant and may be doubly harmful. The chemical (formaldehyde) used to process the special feed which kills the bacteria in the cow's stomach that destroys the essential fatty acids is a known carcinogen. But don't waste time worrying about it. This feed is cost prohibitive and will never catch on.

If you think eliminating cows' milk will cause your teeth to rot and your bones to fail from lack of calcium, I have another surprise for you. The calcium present in cows' milk is in a very heavy form, difficult for the human body to process and assimilate efficiently. In addition, this calcium is mixed up with the protein *casein,* which is the principal amino acid in cheeses and milk curds. Both the calcium and casein in cows' milk are easily digested when they pass through the four stomachs of a baby calf, but have a hard time making their way through the human digestive tract. Cows' milk contains 300 times *more* casein than mothers' milk.

You won't have to worry about a calcium deficiency if you are following the dietary recommendations put forth by the medical authorities cited in this book. The good green leafy vegetables, most fruits, and all nuts are rich sources of easily absorbed calcium. Seeds (raw) are excellent sources of calcium. In fact, sesame seeds are delicate, delicious, and extremely high in quality calcium.

AVOIDABLE CARCINOGENS

TOBACCO — No matter how much the tobacco companies may try to make us believe that there is no conclusive evidence linking tobacco use with cancer, is there anyone out there who still goes along with that desperate line of malarky? It can't be long before the Marlboro man falls off his horse and gasps his last. Because of the documented danger to health posed by smoking, and because more and more smokers are giving up their habit, it can be truly said that — in more ways than one — smokers *are* a dying breed. The harmful effects of smoking have been well publicized. Unless you've been deliberately ignoring the onslaught of information, you know that smoking fosters the development of cancer, heart disease, and more.

K.E. Stanley, Ph.D., of the World Health Organization, publishing in *Cancer Detection & Prevention* (Volume 9:83-89, 1986) points out that over one million premature deaths are caused each year by cigarette smoking. Around the world, lung cancer is the second most common form of malignancy (only stomach cancer accounts for more deaths), with close to 600,000 new cases being diagnosed every year. Between 80 and 90 percent of all lung cancer cases are caused by tobacco. The experts say that the risk is greatest among those who start smoking at a young age and among those who smoke strong, unfiltered cigarettes. Dr. Stanley says, "What is needed now is the implementation of national programs of education and legislation with the objective to establish nonsmoking as the cultural norm. There is probably nothing we could do in the way of prevention that would have a larger impact — not only on cancer incidence, but also on cardiovascular diseases and chronic lung diseases — than eliminating tobacco smoking."

Science says that smoking plays a major part in the development of cancer (lung, bladder, esophagus, mouth, throat), emphysema, bronchial problems, and cardiovascular disease. The most hideous aspect of these often deadly conditions is that they take years to develop. Danger signs usually don't appear until the disease is well along and difficult to treat. Early symptoms that smoking is adversely affecting the body include chronic shortness of breath, excessive tiredness, morning headaches, the typical 'smoker's cough,' hoarseness, diminished circulation resulting in a pale complexion, an impaired sense of taste and smell, prematurely aged skin, and sores and/or tenderness of the gums, tongue, and lips. A smoker is intimately acquainted with these symptoms and usually deals with the problems they create by ignoring them.

When a smoker is forced to quit because of serious illness — or gets smart and decides to give up the habit before early problems escalate into an irreversible condition he will experience some withdrawal symptoms, not as severe as those a drug addict suffers, but just as real. Mild discomfort can include a feeling of dizziness, light-headedness, and drowsiness. Anyone with a real desire to quit can handle these minor symptoms. But the nicotine withdrawal symptom that is hardest to overcome (and live with) is a case of screaming nerves. This is the danger point. It's just so easy to light up and feed the habit.

The smokers among us just can't pretend any longer that they're only hurting themselves either. *Second-hand smoke* is the target of the latest research, resulting in some hard legislative action against smokers all across the country — with good reason.

Great-grandmother used to send great-grandfather out behind the barn when he just had to have a smoke so that her horsehair sofa and the heavy velvet drapes in her front parlor wouldn't reek. She had the right idea, but for the wrong reasons. If a loved one (or co-worker) won't stop smoking for his own good health, and many people won't, he should know that he is endangering the health of the entire family. Inhaling second-hand smoke has been documented as a real health hazard. Studies show that non-smokers breathe in as much of the principle cancer-causing compound in smoke (equivalent to smoking four cigarettes) just by spending one hour in the same room with smokers.

The 'sidestream smoke' which exits directly into the atmosphere from the burning tobacco contains twice the amount of tar and nicotine as is in second-hand smoke (which is 'filtered' through the smoker), and between three and five times as much notoriously harmful elements (cadmium, nitrous oxides, benzopyrene, and carbon monoxide), plus a whopping fifty times as much ammonia as is in the smoke that the smoker himself inhales. Children who live with smokers are triply endangered, first, because they are forced to inhale all those harmful substances; second, because their lungs and bodies are small; and third, because studies show they will most likely become smokers themselves.

If you can't quit for yourself, quit for those you love. After all, you wouldn't deliberately infect a loved one with a terminal disease. Why subject them to the harmful effects of second-hand smoke?

HOW TO QUIT — A few years ago, *aversion therapy* (every puff was accompanied by a mild electric shock) enjoyed a brief vogue, but didn't prove successful over the long term. *Medical hypnosis* continues to be popular, but doesn't eliminate the need for will power. Stop-Smoking programs utilizing a form of *group therapy support* are provided by many hospitals and health organizations. These programs report a high success rate. And, a new nicotine-resin impregnated *chewing gum* (Nicorette) is purported to ease nicotine withdrawal symptoms and help conquer the psychological problems associated with quitting smoking. It cannot be taken by a pregnant or nursing mother and must be prescribed by a physician, but it might be worth talking to your doctor about.

Many successful quitters say that going *cold turkey* and simply stopping smoking all at once works better than anything else. If you are truly addicted, remember that after just 72 hours, the worst will be over. By the end of 5 days, the majority find their craving for nicotine is either eliminated, or is so diminished that it is no longer a problem. In contrast, those who have tried *tapering-off* by consciously reducing the number of cigarettes they smoke daily find it more difficult to make that all-important final break.

For a quick detoxification program that works, you should know that studies have shown that megadoses of Vitamin C, when combined with *cysteine* (an amino acid found abundantly in bee pollen, sunflower and sesame seeds) is able to assist the body in detoxifying nicotine. The B vitamins, plus C and cysteine, also fight the harmful effects of *acetaldehyde,* an irritating element present in tobacco smoke. And, no matter how much you *think* you need a smoke, wait 60 seconds. You may be surprised to find that the craving isn't as strong as you thought. When the urge strikes, practice deep breathing. Smokers are usually shallow breathers who only breathe deeply when they inhale.

A national movement backed by the American Cancer Society, the American Heart Association, and the American Medical Association is aimed at the 30 percent of U.S. adults who are still smokers. You may soon be denied the right to puff away on air flights. A new report by the National Academy of Sciences has determined that the second-hand smoke drifting through the plane from the Smoking Section is harmful to both the crew and non-smoking passengers. Scrapings taken from the air vents shows a heavy concentration of the dangerous pollutants present in tobacco smoke. The problem is compounded because many airlines routinely cut back on the force of their ventilation systems once the plane is off the ground to save fuel, thereby reducing operating costs.

The National Academy of Sciences report has gone to the Transportation Department, accompanied by condemning commentary prepared by the ACS, the AHA, and the AMA. If the legislation is pushed through, smoking may be completely banned on the more than 16,000 domestic flights that cross the country every day. However, the controversy promises to be a lengthy one. The tobacco industry is marshalling its forces, but the medical scientists have a powerful rebuttal ready this time.

SMOKELESS TOBACCO — The practice of dipping snuff and chewing tobacco used to be confined primarily to the rural south. However, for the past few years, tobacco companies have staged a concentrated advertising campaign aimed at our young men. Media ads and television spots featuring sports personalities and entertainers have made a habit which was once considered 'nasty' and 'dirty' into one now thought to be attractive, 'macho,' and less harmful than smoking. Not true.

As a matter of fact, the smokeless tobacco user is at greater risk of developing oral cancer than the smoker. Data developed by the American Cancer Society shows that the risk of developing oral cancer is more than twice as high for the smokeless tobacco addict as for the smoker and that risk increases markedly with long-term exposure. According to statistics from the ACS (Epidemiology & Statistics of Cancer Detection), there were upwards of seven million smokeless tobacco users in the U.S. in 1984 alone. More recent estimates range as high as twenty-two million users, increasing at the terrifying rate of 11 percent every year.

If you or someone you love has been misled into believing that smokeless tobacco is a less harmful form of a proven carcinogen, contact the American Cancer Society and ask for their research reports showing the dangers of smokeless tobacco. ACS has some highly technical material designed to educate health professionals (Cancer Journal for Clinicians), plus some literature (Smokeless Tobacco: Cause for Concern) that is easier reading for the rest of us.

FLUORIDE — *"In point of fact, fluoride causes more human cancer death, and causes it faster, than any other chemical."* So says Dean Burk, Chief Chemist Emeritus of the U.S. National Cancer Institute. As if this statement by a recognized cancer authority isn't damning enough, if you walk into a store to purchase fluoride, it will carry the Skull & Crossbones on its label, the universal symbol for a dangerous poison. In far too many cities across the nation, we are forced to ingest fluoride with our drinking water whether we want to or not. Because this is a free country, we do have several alternatives.

We can go to the expense of purchasing and installing water-purifying equipment that will remove this dangerous carcinogen from our tap water, or we can buy clean water from a delivery service, or we can purchase it by the jug at the store. Of course, we don't like paying several times over for the same product. Not many people can afford to buy clean water for bathing, flushing the commode, and watering the garden, so we have to pay the city water department, *and* we have to pay for drinking and cooking water.

CHEMICALLY-ALTERED FATS — It is an undeniable fact

that the incidence of cancer, heart disease, liver and kidney dysfunction, arthritis, multiple sclerosis, and other conditions of fatty degeneration have risen on a parallel course with our consumption of these heavily-advertised dietary fats. There is just too much hard-won evidence that the body cannot process these chemically altered fats. (See Chapter 5.)

Note: The important health-promoting products mentioned in this chapter should be available in major health food stores nationwide. Each is unique. It's worth searching the stores and wearing out a pair of shoes to find those that seem good to you, but you can order direct from the distributor if you prefer. (See Chapter 16.)

Chapter XIII
Getting Back To Basic Nutrition

A Review of the Four Basic Food Groups

Eating right is very simple. All we really need to do is follow the basic *Dietary Guidelines for Americans,* issued in 1980 by the Department of Health & Human Services, as follows:

- Eat a variety of foods
- Maintain ideal weight
- Avoid the wrong kinds of fat
  - chemically-altered fats, saturated animal fats
- Eat foods with adequate complex carbohydrates & fiber
- Avoid sugar and excessive salt

Ever since kindergarten, when colorful pictures of the four basic food groups were commonly posted around the classroom, we have had it drilled into our consciousness that we should eat a measure of each of the four basic food groups every day. Our dietary needs haven't changed over the years. However, what *have* changed are the ways in which foods are manufactured and processed. Dr. Lendon Smith, M.D. said it best: "If man made it, it's probably dangerous." As you review the following chart, be aware that whole foods, not refined and overprocessed foods, are well represented.

THE FOUR BASIC FOOD GROUPS

Food Group	Servings Daily	One Serving Equals:
Group #1 Fruits & Vegetables	Four	½ cup juice; ½ cup raw (or cooked) vegetable or fruit; portion commonly served, such as one banana, one medium apple or orange
Group #2 Whole-Grains	Four	1 slice of whole-grain bread; ½ cup cooked whole-grain cereal, rice, pasta, grits; 1 cup of whole-grain ready-to-eat cereal
Group #3 Dairy Products	Two	1 cup of milk (low-fat, or skim); 1 cup yogurt (low-fat, unsugared); 2 cups cottage cheese (low-fat); 1½ ounces cheese (natural, unprocessed)
Group #4 Protein Sources	Two	2 ounces fish, poultry, lean meat; Protein Sources ½ cup cottage cheese (low-fat); 2 eggs; 2 ounces hard cheese; ½ cup dried legumes, peas, beans (cooked)

FRUITS & VEGETABLES — Food Group 1

We should eat four or more servings of fruits and vegetables every day. Most authorities recommend that we eat some fresh fruit daily and a dark green or deep yellow vegetable at least every other day. Because some of the important vitamins are lost in cooking, plan to eat at least a portion of your vegetables (and leafy greens) raw, perhaps in a salad. Along with their healthy content of complex carbohydrates and cleansing fiber, fruits and vegetables supply vitamins A, C, and P (the bioflavonoids).

VITAMIN A — This vital fat-soluble vitamin is manufactured in the body from beta-carotene. It is essential for normal growth and development, for maintainenance of the skin (the largest eliminative organ of the body), and for good teeth and bones. A deficiency of vitamin A lowers our resistance to infections, interferes with our ability to adapt to darkness (night blindness), and can affect the cornea of the eye. Healthy hair growth depends on a sufficient supply of vitamin A as well.

The Institute of Cancer Research at Vienna University (Austria) has reported on approximately 1,150 cancer patients treated with megadoses of vitamin A. This vitamin therapy was shown to enhance the effects of radiation and chemotherapy. Even when vitamin A was used alone against squamous cell carcinomas of the skin, the scientists said that a complete remission was obtained. In a series of experiments with lab animals, vitamin A injections (fortified with amygdalin [see Chapter 12] and natural enzymes) brought dramatic results against massive tumors. After four days of intramuscular injections, a pimple appeared at the site of the tumor. Two days later, the pimple broke open and discharged pus. A microscopic examination of the discharge showed the presence of dead tumor cells. As the pus continued to discharge over time, the tumors receded. Four to six weeks later, over 90 percent of the animals were completely free of tumors.

Note: Because megadoses of vitamin A can result in liver dysfunction, a specially prepared water-soluble form of the vitamin was used in the studies reviewed above. High doses of vitamin A cannot be considered a home treatment.

The University of Arizona (Tucson, Arizona) has published research by F.L. Meyskens, Jr., M.D. showing that applying vitamin A to precancerous cells in the cervix of 18 female patients resulted in six cases of remission after just four days of treatment. And scientists at the Albert Einstein College of Medicine (New York) discovered that women showing evidence of early precancerous changes of the cervix commonly ate a diet deficient in beta-carotene, vitamin A, and vitamin C.

Food Sources of Vitamin A — The green and yellow-orange vegetables are rich sources of natural vitamin A, as are many fruits (prunes, pineapples, oranges, limes, and cantaloupes). Other sources of vitamin A include liver, cod liver oil, butter, milk, and egg yolks.

VITAMIN C — Ascorbic acid (vitamin C) is essential for the formation of connective tissue all over the body. It is the inter-cellular 'glue' which maintains the strength of tissues and cells and is vital for strong capillary walls. Evidence suggests that supplying the body with vitamin C in quantity can protect against the common cold. The *Journal of Human Nutrition* (February 1981) tells us that vitamin C can increase the level of high-density lipoproteins (HDL) in the blood. HDL protects against cardiovascular disease. Nobel prize winner Linus Pauling has documented the fact that cancer patients usually exhibit a very low level of ascorbic acid in their infection-fighting white blood cells (leucocytes). Dr. Pauling has also confirmed that cancer patients given high doses of vitamin C live longer and feel better. Statistics show that a diet high in fruits and vegetables can lower the incidence of stomach cancer.

Food Sources of Vitamin C — The citrus fruits are prime sources of vitamin C, but other fruits (strawberries, apples, pears, apricots, plums, peaches, pineapples) are also good. Many vegetables (rutabagas, tomatoes, onions, carrots, green peppers, radishes, carrots, celery, lettuce) offer a healthy content of vitamin C also.

239

VITAMIN P — The bioflavonoids (rutin, hesperidin, citrin) have been collectively dubbed vitamin P, because they exercise a strengthening effect on the permeability of the capillaries, the tiniest blood vessels. Bioflavonoids are essential for the efficient absorption and assimilation of vitamin C. They also work with vitamin C to keep collagen healthy. Collagen represents about 30 percent of the total protein content of the body. It is an important element of cellular connective tissue, promotes youthful elasticity of the skin, and is a vital part of ligaments, cartilage, and bone.

Food Sources of Vitamin P — Fresh fruits and vegetables are good sources of the bioflavonoids, but they are missing in juices and are largely destroyed by cooking. It is the pulpy part (in vegetables and fruits) and thin skin separating the sections in citrus that provides the Vitamin P. Mother Nature always provides vitamin C and vitamin P in the same foods, because each activates the other. Together, they are more potent and powerful than either is alone. (See *Food Sources of Vitamin C* above.)

COMPLEX CARBOHYDRATES — The complex carbohydrates in fruits and vegetables fill you up, but not out. For years, dieters have considered carbohydrate as the villain in a weight-loss regimen, but complex carbos should actually total more than half of the total calories we eat every day. Carbohydrates are the natural fuel (energy) source of the body, but they serve another important function as well. The body converts complex carbohydrates into energy (glycogen) for short-term storage in the liver. This nutrient protects against toxins and controls the breakdown of proteins. Protein can be used for energy production when necessary, but is absolutely vital for cell growth and repair. By supplying the body with complex carbos, we are protected against the nitrogenous waste that is a by-product of the breakdown of proteins.

Food Sources of Complex Carbohydrates — Nature packs complex carbohydrates into just about everything that grows.

In other words, all foods of plant origin are high in the complex carbohydrates essential to life. Remember, it's the *refined* carbohydrates and empty calories present in over-processed manufactured food items that contribute to obesity and many other health problems, not nature's pure version of this important nutrient.

FIBER — The recommendation of the American Cancer Society that we increase our intake of fiber is based on solid research showing that societies which commonly consume a diet high in fiber have a very low incidence of colorectal and intestinal cancers. The difference between these so-called primitive civilizations and our highly industrialized country is primarily one of bowel habits. African natives, for instance, may empty their bowels as often as two or three times every day.

Close to 15 percent of all cancer deaths in this country in 1982, according to the National Cancer Institute (Surveillance, Epidemiology & End Results), were caused by colon and rectal cancers. The body is designed to excrete waste after every meal, but we have come to believe that it's 'normal' to have a bowel movement twice a week. Constipation is a national problem. But certain elements in bile acids can turn into cancer-causing carcinogens. When these carcinogenic substances stay in contact with the colon for a lengthy period, such as when we are constipated, a malignancy can develop. The experts say that simply increasing our intake of fiber, thereby eliminating the constipation factor, can reduce this frightening statistic markedly.

Another factor in favor of fiber is that it is a good source of *silicon*. Silicon occurs in the skeletal structure and teeth, helps maintain the integrity of the arterial system, and assists in strengthening connective tissue all over the body. The experts believe silicon is a preventive against heart disease and arthritis.

Food Sources of Fiber — Of the fruits and vegetables, the best sources of fiber are fresh blackberries, fresh apples, dried figs, dried dates, broccoli, cauliflower, parsnips, pumpkin, and rutabaga. There is another very good source of fiber. See below.

WHOLE GRAINS (BREADS, CEREALS) — Food Group 2

A healthy diet should include four or more servings of whole grain foods every day. Grains are truly the staff of life for most of the world. In the Far East, rice is eaten at every meal. In the Middle East, the cuisine features bulgur (parboiled wheat). We all know (and love) the pasta of Italy. In the Soviet bloc countries, black bread is a delicious and healthy staple. And many of us have become acquainted with the tortillas that are the backbone of the menu south-of-the-border.

But, in America (sometimes called the 'breadbasket of the world'), we often bypass the staff of life. We just don't have a favorite grain that we serve with every meal. Oh, sure, we may give the children a bowl of cereal before sending them off to school. But very often we are serving the 'latest' in a long string of artificially colored 'cereals' (which tint the milk with dye) made popular by colorful (and repetitive) kid-oriented TV commercials. This cereal is probably also over-refined, heavily sugared, and contains many additives.

Whole grain products provide complex carbohydrates, B and E vitamins, iron, magnesium (and traces of other minerals), and more of the healthy fiber we need. The protein in whole grains is incomplete. On a completely vegetarian diet, plant proteins are made complete by eating foods containing the missing amino acids (legumes, milk) at the same meal.

THE B COMPLEX VITAMINS — The water-soluble vitamins known collectively as B Complex include: thiamine (B1), riboflavin (B2), niacin (B3, or nicotinic acid), pyridoxine (B6), biotin, inositol, p-aminobenzoic acid (PABA), cyanocobalamine (B12), pantothenic acid, and folic acid. Medical science has determined that a lack of any one of the Bs brings on a host of medical problems. In other words, we need them all.

The B vitamins affect the growth processes, appetite, the gastro-intestinal tract, the nervous system, the endocrine glands (especially the adrenals), reduce blood sugar levels in diabetes, are necessary for carbohydrate metabolism, and are useful in treating tuberculosis. To give you a grasp of just how important the entire complex of Bs are, consider: A deficiency of B complex can result in an enlarged liver, degeneration of the sex glands, an upset of the nervous system, and can cause a dysfunction of the heart, liver, spleen, kidneys, pituitary, salivary, and adrenal glands.

Food Sources of B Complex — The primary source of the B vitamins are the whole grains and unpolished brown rice. Other sources of one or more of the Bs include Brewer's yeast, legumes, nuts, green vegetables, poultry, eggs, fruits, fish, and meats (pork, liver, beef, and veal). However, it would be unwise in the extreme to use a diet high in meats to get your B complex at the expense of the whole grains. The unhealthy content of saturated fats in meats make them a suspect addition to the menu.

VITAMIN E — Medical science acknowledges that vitamin E is an essential nutrient for man. Over the past decade, many researchers have been studying the action of this antioxidant, known to protect against the harmful development of certain elements which destroy cells. Science has determined that sufficient vitamin E protects against cardiovascular disease (coronary thrombosis, rheumatic heart disease, angina, hypertensive heart disease), phlebitis, supports the immune system, and reduces cramping (menstrual, night cramps, during exercise). Because vitamin E is known to support the immune system, many health authorities believe it is a good addition to the anti-cancer diet as well.

Food Sources of Vitamin E — Good natural sources of dietary vitamin E include wheat germ, whole grains, and soybeans. Additional sources are beans, some fruits and vegetables, and liver. Note: To protect the essential fatty acids (linoleic and linolenic) from oxidation, vitamin E (as a primary natural antioxidant) has been documented as a necessary adjunct to a diet high in polyunsaturates.

IRON — Because iron is essential to the formation of healthy red blood cells (hemoglobin), it is essential to life. Iron is absorbed from food in the small intestines and is transported, via the bloodstream, to bone marrow, where the production of red blood cells is accomplished. As a component of hemoglobin, iron is essential for the transport of oxygen needed for tissue respiration. A lack of iron leads to anemia, retarded development, and low vitality. Iron deficient individuals very often have an abnormally pale complexion.

Food Sources of Iron — Whole wheat, bran, graham, and oatmeal are all excellent sources of iron. Other good sources include almonds, eggs, oysters, soy beans, liver, kidney, many fruits (apricots, currants, dates, oranges, prunes, raisins, rhubarb), and a lot of vegetables (asparagus, beans, cauliflower, celery, chard, dandelions, lettuce, beets, cabbage, cucumbers, parsnips, peppers, peas, potatoes, radishes, tomatoes, turnips, mushrooms).

However, only a fraction of the organic iron present in foods is absorbed by the body. Medical science says that it's necessary to provide from 15 to 30 mg of iron in the diet to be sure that from 1.0 to 4.0 mg will be absorbed.

MAGNESIUM — The healthy human body contains approximately 25 gm of magnesium, most of which is in the bones. Even a small increase in dietary magnesium has been shown to markedly increase bone density. But this white mineral element is also present in the cells, soft tissues, muscles, and in the body fluids. Magnesium is required to activate important enzymes and is associated with the regulation of body temperature, neuromuscular contractions, the metabolism of fats, and the synthesis of proteins. A concentration of this important nutrient (second only to potassium) is found in all cells.

It has been noted that the spinal fluid of hibernating animals contains a high amount of magnesium. It is believed that muscle tremors (and possibly a tendency to convulsions) may be controlled by adding magnesium to the diet. As one of nature's relaxing nutrients, magnesium taken at bedtime promotes healthy sleep. A lack of magnesium can result in erratic or rapid heart beat (implicated in myocardial infarction), low blood pressure, fatigue, mood swings, depression, anxiety, calcium deposits, kidney stones, and even dental problems. Studies show that laboratory animals given feed with less than two parts per million of magnesium sicken and die.

Food Sources of Magnesium — The experts tell us that magnesium is obtained in sufficient quantity in our daily meals — just as long as the menu includes a good measure of the whole grains, fresh fruits, and fresh vegetables. Excellent sources of magnesium include beans, seeds (pumpkin, sesame, sunflower), almonds, and soybeans.

MANGANESE — Manganese is an essential element needed for normal bone development, and it participates in many enzyme reactions as well. It is involved in fat metabolism and protein synthesis, and assists the cells in the production of energy.

A deficiency of manganese is often exhibited by diabetics, epileptics, and myasthenia gravis victims. A lack of this mineral is believed to contribute to some back problems, sterility, dizziness, tinnitus (noises within the ear), lack of coordination, and apathy. As an aid to the diabetic, supplemental manganese can improve glucose tolerance. Because manganese stimulates important neurotransmitters in the brain, it has been demonstrated to improve memory in some cases. Researchers have discovered that male laboratory animals deprived of manganese become sterile; females deprived of manganese lack the maternal instinct and will not care for their young.

Food Sources of Manganese — The whole grains (bran included) are excellent sources of dietary manganese. Additional sources include seeds, nuts, eggs, legumes, the green leafy vegetables, and blueberries.

MOLYBDENUM — An interesting natural phenomenon is that organic foods which offer vitamin C must have molybdenum in order to produce vitamin C. Molybdenum is required to activate certain enzymes. It is an essential trace element in plant growth, where it is used as a catalyst in fixing nitrogeneous proteins. New Zealand researchers have determined that, as an important trace mineral, molybdenum can protect against tooth decay.

Food Sources of Molybdenum — The whole grains offer molybdenum, as do legumes and green leafy vegetables.

POTASSIUM — Potassium is the principal element in intracellular fluid and is of primary importance. A proper balance of potassium, calcium, and magnesium is required for normal heart action and for the conduction of nerve impulses. A potassium deficiency results in a heart dysfunction, marked weakness of the muscles, dizziness, thirst, and mental confusion.

Food Sources of Potassium — Potassium is present in varying levels in many foods, but the best sources of dietary potassium include the cereal grains, dried peas, and dried beans. Additional sources include fresh vegetables, fresh fruits, fresh fish, fresh poultry, nuts, and molasses.

DAIRY PRODUCTS — Food Group 3

Milk contains a generous amount of protein (see Food Group 4) and calcium, plus the vitamins A, B2, B6, and B12 (see Food Group 2), and is usually fortified with vitamin D. Daily requirements as set forth in the government guidelines say: Adults should take 2 cups of milk; children up to 9 years should take 2 to 3 cups; children 9 to 12 (and pregnant women) should take 3 to 4 cups; young adults 12 to 18 (and nursing mothers) should take 4 cups or more. In all the above daily recommendations, the equivalent in milk products may be substituted for all or a portion of the milk. (See Chapter 12 for some drawbacks to the consumption of cows' milk.)

Food Sources of Dairy Products — Other popular dairy products which may be used in place of milk include cottage cheese, yogurt, various cheeses, and even ice cream or ice milk. However, many of these foods are processed with excessive sugar (or artificial sweeteners), chemical additives, and artificial colors (dyes). Please remember to select low-fat dairy products and watch out for the additives.

CALCIUM — Calcium promotes strong teeth and bones, is essential for the functions of the heart, nerves, and muscles, and is also of great importance in regulating the coagulation factor of blood. Calcium is carried in the bloodstream, but unless its companion nutrients (phosphorus, vitamin D) are available in sufficient supply, calcium absorption will not take place.

A deficiency of calcium causes muscle twitching, spasms, and may result in convulsions. It is important to remember that a high fiber diet acts to decrease the body's ability to assimilate calcium and phosphorus (See Food Group 4). This does not mean that we should reduce fiber, but rather we should compensate accordingly by including additional calcium-rich foods in planning daily meals.

Food Sources of Calcium — Milk has come to be accepted as a primary source of dietary calcium, but even better sources include beans, cauliflower, chard, cheese, eggs, kale, molasses, and rhubarb. Science says that a good supply of calcium can be obtained from almonds, beets, bran, cabbage, carrots, celery, dates, figs, kohlrabi, lemons, lettuce, oatmeal, oranges, oysters, parsnips, pineapple, raspberries, rutabagas, shellfish, spinach, turnips, walnuts, and watercress.

VITAMIN D — Because vitamin D is essential in the metabolism of calcium and phosphorus, it is essential for the normal development and maintenance of the skeletal structure and teeth. D is sometimes called the 'sunshine vitamin' because exposure to the sun (or ultraviolet light) synthesizes vitamin D in the body. Without vitamin D, the bones grow soft and/or diseased, rickets develops, and teeth cannot be efficiently remineralized.

Food Sources of Vitamin D — Vitamin D is present in milk (if it has been so enriched), butter, eggs, and fish oils (primarily cod and salmon).

THE PROTEIN SOURCES — Food Group 4

A complete protein is one that contains all the essential amino acids (tryptophane, lysine, methionine, valine, leucine, isoleucine, phenylalanine, threonine, arginine, histidine). Complete protein is essential for growth, the building of new tissue, and the repair of injured or weak tissue. Proteins are used first in the manufacture of red blood cells (hemoglobin), second for the production of blood plasma proteins, and third in tissue repair where needed. Proteins form an integral part of the protoplasm of every cell in the body and are essential to the life processes.

Food Sources of Protein — Because we are traditionally a meat-eating society, the first protein source which springs to mind is meat, especially red meat. However, we must keep the strong recommendation of both the American Cancer Society and the American Heart Association that we reduce our consumption of saturated animal fats firmly in mind when considering the food sources of proteins.

Fish, poultry, eggs, and bee pollen are all excellent sources of rich protein, as are the legumes (beans, peas, lentils, chickpeas), seeds, and nuts. Yes, peanuts are a good source of protein. But commercially processed peanut butters are both sugared and made with partially hydrogenated oils. (See Chapter 5.) Health food stores offer a natural version containing nothing but ground peanuts. Because natural peanut butters are not homogenized, the peanut oil will rise to the top. If you want a peanut butter that comes close to the commercial varieties, you may want to blend in a little honey and a pinch of salt.

COPPER — Copper mates with iron in the manufacture of red blood cells, but about three-quarters of the body's copper is in the bones. Some authorities believe a deficiency of copper is implicated in the development of osteoporosis. It makes a vital contribution to the skeletal structure and helps maintain the integrity of the arterial system. Because so many homes are fitted with copper plumbing, an excess of copper is more common than a deficiency.

Food Sources of Copper — In nature, copper sources include liver, nuts, and oysters.

LECITHIN — Lecithin is one of the 'friendly fats,' shown in research to help hold harmful cholesterol in suspension in the bloodstream, thereby preventing the buildup of the atherosclerotic plaque implicated in heart disease. Lecithin also offers choline (an important amino acid) and steps up the body's production of acetylcholine (a neurotransmitter). Autopsies confirm that acetylcholine is notably low in the brains of Alzheimer's disease victims. The prestigious British medical journal *Lancet* has reported that individuals with Alzheimer's disease (and some forms of learning disabilities) can be helped by adding lecithin to the diet.

Food Sources of Lecithin — The highest concentration of lecithin in nature is found in the yolk of eggs, debunking the medical admonition of some years ago that eating eggs contributes to high cholesterol levels.

PHOSPHORUS — This is another mineral important to the strength and density of bones and teeth, essential in the absorption and utilization of calcium. Phosphorus compounds are the principal sources of energy in muscle contractions, and its presence is required to enable the body to convert glycogen to glucose, our prime source of energy.

Food Sources of Phosphorus — Phosphorus is found in the proteins of food. Excellent sources of phosphorus include almonds, beans, barley, bran, cheese, eggs, lentils, liver, milk, oatmeal, peanuts, peas, walnuts, whole wheat, and rye.

SULFUR — Sulfur is an important element present in every cell of both animals and plants. It is required for the synthesis of proteins and collagen. A deficiency affects the skin and nails, and contributes to both anemia and hair loss. Sulfur works with the B complex vitamins and assists in the efficient metabolism of the essential fatty acids.

Food Sources of Sulfur — Cottage cheese (low-fat) is a primary source of the sulfur-rich proteins (recommended in conjunction with linseed oil [see Chapter 6] by Dr. Johanna Budwig). Many other foods contain sulfur, including eggs, peanuts, onions, garlic, and whole cereal grains.

ZINC — The breast milk of a new nursing mother contains a strong concentration of zinc for the first two weeks, with a sharp drop noted after that period. A newborn child's liver contains three times as much zinc as the liver of an adult, showing that nature considers this mineral vital for normal development. Zinc is always present in human tissues, but the greatest concentration occurs in the thyroid and sex organs at adulthood. Zinc contributes to a wide variety of bodily functions, but requires the help of vitamin A. It is vitamin A which mates with zinc stored in the liver. Zinc and vitamin A are commonly given together for the treatment of acne, eczema, and psoriasis.

A study conducted at Purdue University (Lafayette, Indiana) determined that close to 60 percent of adult Americans over the age of 60 lack zinc. Early symptoms of a zinc deficiency include a measurable loss of taste and smell, and wounds that heal poorly and slowly. Other research has shown that the blood of rheumatoid arthritis victims is markedly lacking in zinc. When zinc was replaced in the diet, the arthritic patients reported less early morning stiffness, less swelling of joints, and found they could walk for a longer period of time without pain. Health authorities say that a severe zinc deficiency contributes to cancer, cystic fibrosis, low sperm count in males, prostatitis, a loss of libido, menstrual problems in the female, and toxemia during pregnancy. In medically prescribed doses of 100 mg daily, zinc has been shown to increase the production of antibodies.

Food Sources of Zinc — The natural zinc in foods is almost completely destroyed in commercial food processing. To add to the problem, the zinc content of the soil in most agricultural states has been exhausted. The experts say that a good diet should include approximately 15 mg of zinc daily. The best sources are liver (3 ounces yields 6 mg of zinc), and peanut butter (3 ounces yields 3 mg of zinc).

WHAT'S MISSING FROM THE FOUR BASIC FOOD GROUPS?

ESSENTIAL FATTY ACIDS — There is a vast quantity of material in this book showing the important functions of the essential fatty acids (linoleic and linolenic). Remember, 'essential' means just that. The body cannot manufacture linoleic or linolenic fatty acids from other elements. They must be supplied daily in the diet. (See Chapters 5 & 6.)

Food Sources of the Essential Fatty Acids — There has been quite a bit written lately about the benefits of olive oil and salmon oil. While both are good sources of fatty acids, neither one contains both linoleic and linolenic fatty acids. The best sources of the essential fatty acids in human nutrition are linseed oil, soybean oil, pumpkin oil, and walnut oil. Only these four oils, and *only when they are not altered in processing,* offer both essential fatty acids. Please see chart below.

ESSENTIAL FATTY ACIDS CONTENT OF COMMON VEGETABLE OILS

Source	Fat Content Total %	Essential Fatty Acids Linolenic	Linoleic	Both Essentials Total %
Linseed	35	58	14	72
Soybean	18	9	50	59
Pumpkin	47	15	42	57
Walnut	60	5	51	56
Rapeseed*	30	7	30	37
Safflower	59	0	75	
Sunflower	47	0	65	
Grape	Trace	0	71	
Corn	4	0	59	
Wheat Germ	10	0	54	
Sesame	49	0	54	
Rice Bran	10	0	35	
Cotton**	Trace	0	50	
Peanut***	47	0	29	
Almond	54	0	17	
Macadamia	71	0	10	
Cashew	41	0	6	
Olive	20	0	8	
Coconut	35	0	3	
Palm Kernel	35	0	3	

*   Rapeseed (canola) contains toxic *erucic acid*

**   Cottonseed contains common toxins

*** Peanuts (damp) harbor a toxic fungus

Hemp (not listed because it is illegal in the U.S.)

provides both essential fatty acids

SELENIUM — This powerful antioxidant has been shown in scientific research to inhibit the formation of tumors, probably by stimulating the production of important antibodies. Lab animals first given selenium and then deliberately exposed to toxic chemicals were found to have developed a degree of immunity to the toxins. The National Cancer Institute has said that just 200 mcg (micrograms) of selenium daily might be a cancer preventive. Based on on-going animal and human studies, the experts are saying that cancer rates across the board could be decreased over the long term by as much as 70 percent if the general population merely ingested this small of amount of selenium daily. Japanese women, who commonly consume a diet which provides from 250 to 350 mcg of selenium daily, have a very low rate of breast cancer, just one-fifth that of American women.

Food Sources of Selenium — Natural dietary selenium has become difficult to find. As long ago as 1965, studies showed conclusively that persons living in areas where selenium was present in strong concentration in the soil and water enjoyed a lower rate of cancer than the national average. Unfortunately, some chemical fertilizers (sulfates) inhibit selenium development in food crops, and the soil in a vast number of states is deficient (or totally devoid) of selenium.

Foods grown in North Dakota, South Dakota, and/or Nebraska still offer a good content of natural selenium. If you live in these states and/or eat foods grown in these states, you're in luck. For the rest of us, an alternative to consider is the fact that *Desert Gold Crown*™ *Bee Pollen,* a comprehensive blend of pollens harvested in the Dakotas and other western states, provides a healthy amount of natural selenium. (See Chapter 9.)

NUTRITION AND HEALTH

If you're still not convinced that what we eat controls how we feel and the degree of health we enjoy, here's what some medical scientists and recognized health authorities have found.

Kanematsu Sugiura, M.D., a researcher at the Sloan-Kettering Cancer Institute, discovered a few years ago that *amygdalin,* a natural substance found in many seeds and nuts, better known as laetrile or B17 (see Chapter 12) is a powerful inhibitor of cancer. Dr. Sugiura's report states, "Amygdalin caused regression (of tumors) in 80 percent of the animals studied, and complete regression in 40 percent. There is a significant inhibition of the formation of lung metastases and it possibly prevents, to an uncertain degree, the formation of new tumors." Sloan-Kettering suppressed Dr. Sugiura's report and discontinued research on the properties of amygdalin.

Another nutrient source which showed great promise in early testing as a natural cancer inhibitor was bee pollen. (See Chapter 9.) U.S. government studies (Department of Agriculture) investigating the benefits of bee pollen were dropped with no explanation.

Important research conducted by A.B. Robinson, Ph.D. at the Linus Pauling Institute (Menlo Park, California) shows conclusively the part diet plays in conquering cancer. After inducing cancer in laboratory animals, Group 1 was given a diet consisting only of apples, bananas, carrots, pears, sunflower seeds, tomatoes and wheat grass. Group 2 was given very high vitamin C (along with commercially manufactured feed). Group 3 was given high vitamin C in addition to the same raw diet fed to Group 1. The results were definitive. In the animals in Group 1 and Group 2, the cancerous lesions were reduced five-fold. But in Group 3, given both the raw diet *and* high vitamin C, an astounding and very satisfying 35-times decrease in cancerous lesions was achieved. Dr. Robinson points out, "The incidence of severe cancerous lesions in these experiments was caused to vary over a 70-fold range by *nutritional measures alone."*

Albert Schweitzer, physician, humanitarian, and winner of the Nobel Peace Prize in 1952, was astounded to discover a completely cancer-free society on his arrival in French Equatorial Africa in 1913. Dr. Schweitzer wrote: "I was astonished to encounter no cases of cancer. I saw none among the natives 200 miles from the coast. This absence of cancer seems to be due to the difference in *nutrition of the natives,* as compared to the Europeans."

253

From 1942 to 1946, a steady decrease in the number of dental caries (cavities) was documented in the population of Norway. The reason? Food rationing during World War II took sugar and other refined carbohydrates off the market. In place of refined over-processed foods, Norwegians were taking vegetables, bread, potatoes, and milk. By 1947, the eating of refined foods had returned to pre-war levels and the incidence of dental problems kept pace.

As long ago as 1944, an article by Dr. H.H. Turner published in the *Pennsylvania Medical Journal* pointed out that close to 90 percent of the adults over age 45 had vision problems. Dr. Turner expressed his belief that the carbonic acid found in carbonated soft-drinks (sodas), devoured in large quantities by a huge percentage of the population, was responsible for the great increase in near-sightedness (myopia) in the U.S.

"America is one of the sickest and worst fed nations on earth." So states J.C. Nichols, M.D., a noted medical writer. Dr. R.J. Williams, professor of biochemistry, the University of Texas (Austin, Texas), states without equivocation, "Enumerating various changes characteristic of aging (impaired vision, hearing, memory, strength and endurance decline, insomnia, loss of libido and appetite for food, aches and pains, increased tendency toward constipation, arthritis, diabetes, arteriosclerosis, osteoporosis, senility, etc.), I want to call attention to the idea that every one of the cells and tissues in the body have to perform their functions properly and also that every one of these failures is related to *cell and tissue nutrition*. We can state with assurance that the longer cells are furnished with the necessities of life, including good nutrition, the longer they will continue to remain in good working order."

The dietary recommendations of the American Cancer Society (and the American Heart Association), reviewed and thoroughly explained in this book, have refined the basic guidelines given above even further. The Director of the National Cancer Institute's prevention program, Dr. Peter Greenwald, has been quoted as saying, "Laboratory studies suggest certain vitamins have an inhibitory effect on cancer."

We remind you that cells and the products of cells form all the tissues of the body. All functions of the body are carried on by cells, both individually and collectively. Cells arise only from preexisting cells by a process of cell division. Growth and development occur from an increase in the numbers of cells and the differentiation of cells into different types of tissues. It is obvious that if we keep the cells in good working order by supplying them with the nutrients they require to proceed with the life processes, we are then practicing a very effective form of preventive medicine indeed.

Chapter XIV
Looking Ahead To The Year 2000?

Can We Cut The Cancer Death Rate in Half by 2000?

After two decades of intensive research and data collection, The National Cancer Institute says we have the knowledge to reduce the mortality rate of cancer by fifty percent (or more) by the beginning of the next century. That's less than fifteen years into the future — within the lifetime of most of us — and certainly well within the lifetime of our children. This isn't space-age fiction coming from the pen of a talented science fiction writer either. Serious scientists and oncologists, a group not noted for their impetuosity or optimism, agree that the time has come to embark on a grand and serious crusade to put the knowledge we have gained into practice and take steps to eradicate the killer once and for all.

The NCI tells us that they have accumulated considerable scientific evidence showing that the choices we make when planning the family menu have a lot to do with the development of certain types of cancer. The NCI hammers home the point that smoking is a prime cause of many cancers. Lifestyle, environmental factors, and exposure to carcinogens in the workplace are targeted by the NCI as areas where we need to become more aware about the added risk of cancer. Joseph W. Cullen, Ph.D., of the Division of Cancer Prevention & Control, National Cancer Institute, (National Institute of

Health, Bethesda, Maryland), says emphatically, "Epidemiologists have estimated the percentage of U.S. cancer deaths that might be avoided by eliminating some of the known or suspected cancer risk factors — and have stressed that *cancer is largely an avoidable disease when adequate preventive measures are taken.*

Dr. Cullen continues, "Tobacco use and dietary habits constitute the greatest risk factors for cancer. Approximately 30 percent of current U.S. cancer deaths might be due to tobacco use. Although the influence of diet on the development of cancer is currently not as clearly defined as for tobacco, epidemiologists assert that it might be possible to avoid as much as 35 percent of cancer deaths by making appropriate changes in dietary habits." The following chart, prepared by the NCI from current data, shows estimates of the avoidable cancer deaths.

PERCENTAGE OF AVOIDABLE CANCER DEATHS

Dietary Factors	**35%**
Tobacco	**30%**
Viruses	**5%**
Occupation	**4%**
Alcohol	**3%**
Excessive Sun	**3%**
Environmental Pollution	**2%**
Food Additives	**1%**
Medicine & Medical Procedures	**1%**

LIFESTYLE FACTORS

In support of the presumption that lifestyle choices influence the development of cancer are studies of two well-known religious groups, both of which follow strict dietary practices and whose members neither smoke nor drink. The state of Utah, home of the Mormons (The Church of Jesus Christ of Latter Day Saints), has consistently enjoyed the lowest incidence of cancer death of all the U.S. states for more than a hundred years. The Mormons do not drink alcohol, coffee, or tea, do not use tobacco in any form, enjoy sex in the marriage bed only, take only moderate amounts of meat, and generally favor a diet of whole foods (with strong emphasis on whole grains, fruits, and vegetables) over refined and over-processed foods.

The rate of cancer mortality for non-smoking Mormon males from the cancers tagged as smoking-related (lungs, esophagus, pharynx, bronchus, trachea, bladder) is 26 percent, the same as for typical non-Mormon nonsmokers. The standardized mortality ratios for cancers not related to the use of tobacco are around 70 percent for male Mormons and around 80 percent for female Mormons, but typical nonsmokers outside this religious group have a risk factor of 100 percent. Overall, the cancer rate for Mormons as a group is 20 to 30 percent *less* than the rate for typical nonsmokers as a group. Obviously, even with tobacco use eliminated, other healthy lifestyle choices are a big factor in the lower rate of cancer mortality enjoyed by the Mormons as a group.

The Seventh-Day Adventists are another religious group which practices a healthy lifestyle. The diet of Seventh-Day Adventists includes no alcohol, caffeinated beverages, or excessively spiced foods. Up to 50 percent of the membership are lacto-ovo (milk and egg) vegetarians and the remainder take little meat. Tobacco use is expressly prohibited. The risk of developing smoking-related lung cancer is a low 17 percent for Seventh-Day Adventist males (34 percent for females), compared to a risk factor of 40 percent for the general non-smoking males (59 percent for females). Overall, cancer mortality from all forms of malignancy is just 53 percent for Seventh-Day

Adventist males (68 percent for females), compared again against the 100 percent risk of the general population.

After adding up the odds, the NCI has come to the conclusion that the low cancer death rate enjoyed by these two religious groups is based on their healthy lifestyle choices. These studies form the basis for the cancer prevention strategies developed by the NCI which they believe will result in a 50 percent reduction in cancer mortality by the year 2000. In his recent report entitled, "Design of Cancer Prevention Studies," Dr. Cullen says, "The NCI has committed itself to an expanded and more aggressive research and control program. This commitment is evidenced by the adoption of a national goal to reduce cancer mortality by 50 percent by the year 2000, the achievement of which is predicated on:

- The aggressive promotion and widespread application of state-of-the-art methods for cancer prevention and management, and
- The tracking of research to identify and evaluate new results ready for application by 1990 and the timely transfer of these results into practice.

"With the means at hand to prevent up to 75 percent of the cancers that currently afflict Americans, the NCI anticipates that realization of this goal will save about 200,000 lives per year. In addition to the approximately 105,000 lives that can be saved each year through wider application of improved detection and treatment techniques, another 95,000 lives can be saved through preventive measures.

"The emphasis of the national cancer prevention strategy is the eradication of the tobacco and dietary influences that contribute to 65 percent of cancer deaths."

THE NCI HAS A PLAN

The NCI has undergone a massive reorganization in the implementation of their avowed goal of reducing cancer deaths by the year 2000. Important groups, with specific responsibilities, have been developed and are already in place and acting. These groups, with their areas of focus, are listed on the next page:

- *The National Steering Committee:* This group coordinates national planning. It helps various agencies on the federal, state, and local levels implement the educational, preventive, and screening programs that will make the goal a reality.
- *National Planning Committees on Prevention, Screening, Detection, Treatment, & Surveillance:* The four groups under this heading, each with a specific area of responsibility, are in the process of developing effective strategies in their respective areas.
- *National Coalition on Cancer Control:* This group is responsible for the development of cancer control programs on a national level. In support of the NCI's goal for the year 2000, it is also responsible for making sure that all data and information is promptly available where needed.
- *NCI Operating Committee:* The Operating Committee oversees all program planning and monitors the day-to-day operations of all programs.
- *NCI Core Planning Team:* Once the initial strategies have been developed, this important group has the responsibility for putting the programs and activities into practice.

Areas targeted by the NCI for development include cancer control programs which focus on the need for prevention, detection and diagnosis, treatment, surveillance, and the development of additional resources. The NCI is taking dead aim against smoking, is actively promoting a preventive diet offering good nutrition, is working to increase the public's awareness of the need for regular screening (especially for breast and cervical cancers), is encouraging the formation of clinical cooperative groups, community clinical oncology programs, and cancer centers, and continues to monitor the SEER (Surveillance Epidemiology and End Results) program. Of prime importance with the focus on cancer prevention are the following aims:

- Reduce smoking by 1990 to half of the 1980 level by:
  - An increasingly active campaign to educate the public to the dangers of tobacco, and

— By the development of quit-smoking (cessation) programs for the hard-core smokers

• Implement additional controlled dietary studies (chemoprevention) to determine the preventive effects of certain micronutrients and macronutrients (fat and fiber).

• Intensify diet and nutritional educational programs aimed at the general public and health professionals alike on the importance of reducing fat and increasing fiber in the diet.

THE NCI vs TOBACCO

The tobacco industry has a real fight on its hands this time. The NCI points out that studies too numerous to count have shown that tobacco use markedly increases the risk of developing cancer. Dr. Cullen says, "Evidence indicates that if large numbers of the population stop smoking (or never begin smoking), the lung cancer death rate in this country could be reduced sharply (instead of steadily increasing) and the total cancer mortality would substantially decline." The NCI has established a five-part program designed to eliminate tobacco use as a cancer risk factor, as follows:

• *Basic Research:* Scientific investigation of the biomedical, epidemiologic, and socio- and biobehavioral aspects of tobacco use, especially studies of the role of smoking and tobacco use in carcinogenesis.

• *Intervention Research:* Research on the modification of tobacco use behavior through the environment, the health care system, or the individual. Whether or not cancer prevention is achievable depends on what individuals do with information about tobacco use as a risk factor for cancer.

• *Information Dissemination:* Development, synthesis, and communication of information about the cancer risk of smoking and tobacco use and the means of reducing that risk. Effective information exchange and dissemination are essential for cancer control.

- *Surveillance & Evaluation:* Monitoring the patterns and trends of cancer-related tobacco use and progress in preventing and controlling such use. This activity makes it possible to identify new populations for targeted interventions, determine the appropriateness and timeliness of intervention studies, and track progress toward accomplishment of established goals and objectives for smoking and tobacco-related cancer control.

- *Liaison:* Coordination of the scientific aspects of STCP (Smoking, Tobacco, & Cancer Program) activities with other federal and nonfederal organizations involved in related efforts through direct collaboration on projects of mutual interest with other sponsoring agencies or through informing other organizations of the general direction and progress of the program.

INTERVENTION — The NCI is looking for ways which can potentially modify behavior and thereby cut down on smoking and the use of other forms of tobacco. In combination, these programs are expected to influence close to five million tobacco users, with around 300,000 receiving full intervention and approximately four and one half million receiving partial intervention. The intervention approaches the NCI believes will prove most effective include:

- *School-Based Educational Programs*
  — to reduce the number of beginning smokers and to encourage students already smoking to quit

The NCI says that data indicates that school-based intervention programs (peer-led programs, films and videotapes, life and social skills training, health-promotion activities, family involvement) does lead to at least short-terms reductions in smoking among students. The NCI says that the number of students receiving programs or follow-up evaluation through funded grants totals around 170,000 to date. Determination of the long-term results of these types of programs is in the works.

Because most smokers begin in their teens, the NCI believes that preventing the habit among the youth of the nation is of prime importance in controlling smoking behavior. Data shows that 15 percent of U.S. teenagers between the ages of 12 and 17 were regular smokers in 1982. The NCI says that every day, 4,000 young people under the age of 17 start smoking. To date, a total of 178,660 teenagers are enrolled in intervention programs and close to 100,000 more are exposed to media messages.

- *Self-Help Programs*
  - to encourage smokers to quit

Studies show that most of the approximately 33 million people who have given up smoking since 1964 did it without help. Smokers say they would rather quit on their own than with the aid of organized cessation programs. The NCI has mounted studies to find out the effectiveness of individual and/or group self-help programs to prevent or stop cigarette smoking, and to find out if going to the expense of developing such programs will be effective over the long-term.

- *Doctors and Dentists*
  - asking health professionals to take a more active part in the prevention of tobacco-related cancers, both in identifying and diagnosing early cancers and in counseling patients on the dangers of tobacco

Recent British studies indicate that health professionals (who are authority figures in most of our lives) can be of immeasurable help in influencing their patients. The British researchers determined that, in a three-minute counseling session initiated by the physician, over five percent of the patients thus encouraged were able to quit smoking and have remained nonsmokers.

Statistics show that there are 380,000 practicing physicians and 135,000 practicing dentists in the U.S. who are viewed by smokers as important factors in their decision to quit smoking. If physicians were successful in encouraging only 4 percent of their patients to quit smoking, approximately 1.4 million smokers would give up the habit every year. Unfortunately, the NCI says that the total number of physicians who are trained in effective methods of counseling their patients against smoking is 700.

- *Mass Media*
  - using effective publicity against smoking

On the plus side, the mass media reaches a great many people at one time; these messages give smokers information on where to find help to quit; and they create a support system which can lead to the necessary changes in behavior. To find out the true effectiveness of the mass media approach, the NCI is doing extensive follow-up studies to see how well this type of intervention is working over the long-term.

- *Policy Intervention*
  - working to establish nonsmoking as the norm

Data regarding tobacco production and consumption, agricultural production, demographics, health, taxation, employment, health care costs, and tobacco production costs are expected to be utilized. The NCI says strong evidence exists showing that smoking intervention programs are more successful when social and economic systems encourage nonsmoking behavior.

POPULATION GROUPS AT RISK — In order to efficiently design intervention programs that work, the NCI has divided certain segments of the population into categories. The groups targeted include:

Women Smokers: In the period from 1950 to 1980, the number of lung cancer deaths among women has increased by more than 700 percent, double the rate of increase documented among men. Statistics show that close to 2,000 teenaged females take up the habit every day. Given this fact, it is hardly surprising to find that lung cancer has begun to overtake breast cancer as the most common cancer among women. The NCI points out that the number of women smokers is about ten years behind that of men. The NCI considers now to be the ideal time to implement intervention programs that take into consideration the smoking patterns unique to women.

Heavy Smokers: The possibility of dying of cancer increases markedly with the number of cigarettes smoked. Those who typically smoke two or more packs of cigarettes every day are multiplying their risk of developing lung cancer by 15 to 25 times. The NCI is currently engaged in examining strategies to entice heavy smokers into quit-smoking programs.

Smokeless Tobacco Users: As recently as 1975, only four percent of the U.S. population were using chewing tobacco and snuff. Today, due to an aggressive advertising campaign, teenagers, young adults, sports figures, and even white collar workers are finding smokeless tobacco very attractive. Studies show that smokeless tobacco use is linked to oral and pharyngeal cancer, plus oral leukoplakia and gum disease. The NCI is currently correlating data and working on intervention programs that will be tested shortly.

Minority Groups: Data shows that tobacco-related cancers (lung, esophagus, larynx) are higher among U.S. blacks than among other minority groups. Many blacks are blue-collar workers and blue-collar workers (of all nationalities) appear to smoke more than those in other professions, resulting in the statistically higher rate of lung cancer exhibited by laborers as a general group. Tobacco-related cancers are currently lower among Hispanics than among blacks or whites, but the latest studies show that Hispanic youths are beginning to smoke cigarettes at a much higher rate than young people of other nationalities. The NCI says that special intervention programs aimed at blacks and Hispanics are needed.

At the current time, approximately 70,000 Hispanics have signed up for community intervention programs. Two and one half million more have been exposed to intensive messages in the media. The NCI says that this total number will be substantially increased as soon as grants focusing on both blacks and Hispanics have been funded.

IMPORTANT DIETARY ADVICE FROM THE NCI

The NCI estimates that approximately 35 percent of all cancers are related to diet. While noting that the complexity of nutritional components makes pinpointing the actual percentage almost impossible, the NCI says that high-fat intake increases the risk of cancer, while high-fiber intake, the vitamins A, C, and E, and selenium are effective dietary preventives against cancer. In the area of cancer prevention, the NCI is concentrating on researching dietary fat, dietary fiber, food composition, modification of eating behavior, and the effects of retinoids and carotenoids.

DIETARY FAT — The NCI says that cancer of the breast, colon, rectum, prostate, and endometrium are promoted by dietary fat. Studies show that breast cancer, in particular, occurs with more frequency among women who eat higher levels of fats (animal fats, saturated or unsaturated fats); who favor fried foods; and those who eat more beef, port, creams, and desserts. In addition, clinical studies show that the survival rate after breast cancer can be positively influenced by a low-fat diet.

Because dietary studies, case control studies, and animal research all show a high relationship between diet and breast cancer deaths, the NCI has mounted studies of humans for the first time. The NCI expects to show that a diet including only 15 percent fat can result in a 25 percent reduction in the occurrence of breast cancer. The typical American diet currently includes 40 percent calories from fat.

DIETARY FIBER — The NCI says that the protective effect of fiber against cancer apparently results because fiber increases stool bulk (thereby effectively diluting the concentration of cancer-causing elements in the stool), and by promoting frequent bowel movements (which moves toxins through the system and out where they can do no harm).

The NCI is working to discover exactly which of the various components of fiber (cellulose, lignin, hemicelluloses, pentosans, gums, pectins) have the greatest preventive effect. Studies are underway to determine the physiochemical effects of fiber in humans and to develop conclusive data on the fraction components of dietary fiber in the human diet.

MODIFYING EATING BEHAVIOR — Most of us select foods that taste good and give no thought to nutritional values. Dr. Cullen points out that, "Avoidance of certain foods can create a conflict between healthful choices and immediate taste satisfactions." The National Academy of Sciences dietary guidelines recommend we avoid foods high in fat, sugar, and salt, while increasing our consumption of fruits, vegetables, and whole-grain products.

The NCI is studying methods of increasing our awareness of the long-range health benefits of eating correctly, but says that the factors which affect our patterns of food selection have not been identified. Dr. Cullen says that, "Interdisciplinary behavioral and nutritional research has been initiated to develop and test such methods within populations at high risk for colon and breast cancer. This research will enhance our understanding of the behavioral aspects of food choices and eating behavior."

RETINOIDS & CAROTENOIDS — The dietary intake of retinoids (vitamin A) and carotenoids (precursors of vitamin A) has been shown to exert a protective effect against cancer. What is not yet clear is exactly which element is most effective. The NCI has studies planned which will analyze the effects of these substances on human metabolism and physiology.

CHEMOPREVENTION — This rather forbidding and high-sounding medical term simply means that certain nutrients have been shown to inhibit the development of cancer. This newly-named area of research is strongly supported by a growing body of evidence that indicates that certain nutrients can slow down cancer growth in various stages of development. Epidemiological studies support the fact that persons eating a diet high in various micronutrients have a much lower incidence of breast, colon, and uterine cancers. Animal studies show that the occurrence of skin, breast, and bladder cancers can be reduced by dietary intake of certain important micronutrients, including the retinoids and carotenoids.

Dr. Cullen says that, "Whereas dietary modification requires acceptance and compliance, the addition of micronutrients to foods is believed to be an easier mechanism through which to effect a reduction in cancer incidence." The NCI is currently studying micronutrients and expects to develop effective non-toxic (or with acceptable low levels of toxicity) chemopreventive agents which can then be applied in a human intervention trial program.

The chemopreventive agents under study include: 4-hydroxy-phenyl retinamide, retinyl acetate, vitamins B6, B12, C, and E, wheat bran, 13-cis retinoic acid, B-carotene, retinol, retinyl palmitate, and sodium selenite. Groups at high risk are being targeted for trials, including: persons with bladder cancer, breast cancer, cervical dysplasia, familial polyposis, adenomatous polyps, basal cell carcinoma, actinic keratoses, chronic smokers, smoking males, persons exposed to asbestos, albinos, and physicians and dentists.

In all, four kinds of chemoprevention human intervention trials are being conducted by the NCI. They are:

- *General Population Studies*
  - A randomized double-blind trial involving 22,000 U.S. physicians has been mounted to evaluate the possible contribution of B-carotene to a decrease in total cancer incidence
- *Studies of High Risk Groups*
  - Heavy smokers (a high-risk group) are being studied to determine the impact of B-carotene in lung cancer
  - Asbestos workers (a high-risk group) are being studied to determine if the dietary intake of B-carotene and retinol is related to lung cancer and mesotheliomas
- *Studies of Patients with Precancerous Lesions*
  - Retinoids are being administered topically to women with mild to moderate cervical dysplasia to determine if retinoids can prevent precancerous lesions from becoming malignant
- *Studies of Prevention of New Primaries in Cancer Patients*
  - The oral administration of B-carotene, 13-cis-retinoic acid, and vitamin A is being studied to determine effectiveness against the development of new cancer sites in existing cancer patients

THE NCI FAVORS A PREVENTIVE APPROACH

It's hard to fault the conclusions reached by Dr. Cullen in this important landmark report. Strong documentation from serious oncologists and scientists around the world, well represented and reported on throughout this entire book, leads us inescapably to the conclusion that the preventive approach is the workable approach. Preventing cancer *is* our best hope for beating this killer.

We close this chapter with a final quote from Dr. Cullen: "The evidence that is currently available about the cancer risks of smoking and diet provides a firm basis for prevention and indicates the need for continued rigorous research. In addition to the NCI's expanded intervention research program, we have launched a major cancer prevention awareness program designed to increase public knowledge of cancer risks, improve public attitudes toward cancer prevention, and influence individuals to modify their behaviors to reduce their risk of cancer. Collectively, the preventive measures undertaken by the NCI provide a significant force for reducing the cancer burden of the American people."

Chapter XV

Forewarned Is Forearmed

*"That man is wise who gains his wisdom
from the experience of another."*

Titus Maccius Plautus, a Roman philosopher and playwright
who lived from 254 to 184 B.C., penned those words over two
thousand years ago. They are as fresh and true today as they
were when the Roman empire ruled the world. Given the fact
that killing disease rampages through our modern and civilized
society today, perhaps they are even more pertinent to our time
than to that of Plautus.

This book is rich in the experiences of others. We have
presented the research of medical scientists world-wide and
detailed some remarkable stories of ordinary people who have
followed healthful regimens which many times brought them
back from the edge of the grave itself. Science *is* making progress, but very slowly, against cancer. But what we must not
do is wait complacently for a cure. We cannot afford to rest
securely in the arms of medical science thinking that a cure
will be found in time to save us. The following facts will show
you very graphically exactly why:

PREVENTION IS VITAL

TESTING THE STATISTICS — Three prestigious medical
research institutions (The Sloan-Kettering Cancer Center, The
Mayo Clinic, and Johns Hopkins University) collaborated in

a study of over 30,000 middle-aged men who were heavy smokers and therefore considered at risk of developing lung cancer. This research involved intensive and regular screening of half the men, with the other half serving as the control group.

To no one's surprise, the screened group had a lot more lung cancer. Because the malignancies were discovered in their very early stages, the patients were immediately put into treatment and showed an excellent survival rate. But, when the data provided by the control group was programmed into the study, it was found that the number of men who died of lung cancer in both the control group and the group diagnosed and treated resulted in virtually identical survival rates.

On the other hand, the early diagnosis and treatment of breast cancer *does* improve the odds for women over the age of fifty, but not for younger women. Under the auspices of the Health Insurance Plan of Greater New York, a 20-year study of 62,000 women (aged 40 to 64) involved offering half the women free annual mammograms and physical examinations, with the other half of the group serving as the control. Far fewer deaths as a result of breast cancer were tabulated in women over age 50 (but not in the younger women) in the group offered free exams than in the control group.

Note: Although no clinical trials have been mounted to determine the usefulness of the vaginal PAP smear, most authorities agree that this test, leading to early diagnosis and treatment, would prove to be of vital importance in increasing survival rates for women.

THE MORTALITY RATE — In 1962, the total cancer mortality rate in the U.S. was 170 persons in every 100,000. In 1982, twenty years later and the latest year for which overall cancer mortality statistics are currently available, the total figure was 185 victims in every 100,000 persons. John Bailar of the Harvard School of Public Health says, "The fundamental problem is not that cancer treatment is ineffective, but that it is not getting better. The figures cited above show why we're worried. Overall cancer mortality is going up."

ANNUAL DEATHS FROM CANCER PER 100 MILLION AMERICANS UNDER AGE 65

Number of Deaths (Male)

30,000 25,000 20,000 15,000 10,000 6,000 2,000 0

Number of Deaths (Female)

0 2,000 6,000 10,000 15,000 20,000 25,000 30,000

Site of Cancer

Legend:
Nonsmokers ▬▬▬
1950s □□□□
1960s ‑‑‑‑
1970s ●●●●

Oral Cancer (mouth, esophagus, larynx)

Lung Cancer

Stomach Cancer

Intestines (including rectum)

Liver, Gallbladder & Bile Ducts

Pancreas

Bone

Skin Cancer

Breast Cancer

Bladder

Kidneys

Prostate

Uterine Cancer (cervix)

Uterine Cancer (endometrium)

Uterine Cancer (ovaries)

Brain & Nervous System

Leukemia

Hodgkin's Disease

Other

PREVENTION *IS* VITAL — With discouraging statistics like these and the mortality rate from cancer continually creeping upward, there's no question whatsoever but that we must protect ourselves and our loved ones from this killer with every means at our disposal.

FOREWARNED IS FOREARMED

NO ONE CAN DO IT FOR YOU — It has become increasingly obvious that we all have some hard choices to make, but *the guideposts are clearly marked.* You can opt to follow a crooked path with many indulgences and heedless diversions along the way. Or you can examine your lifestyle and decide instead to make whatever changes are necessary to put some of the documented preventives to work for you. It's up to you to choose the road you wish to travel.

Health is the natural state of the body. If you make the right choices *now,* all the evidence promises that the quality of life you can enjoy into your sunset years will be rich with both mental and physical pleasures long past three score years and ten.

Here's to your very good health.

William L. Fischer

Chapter XVI
For Your Convenience

Although most of the consumer products discussed in *How To Fight Cancer And Win* are available in major health food stores nationwide, you may sometimes have trouble locating a particular item that seems just right for you.

When that time comes, or if you just plain prefer arm-chair shopping convenience, we suggest you request a catalog from *Biowell*. (Health food retailers, take note. *Biowell* distributes to health food stores all over the U.S.) This forward-thinking organization carries many hard-to-find health-related products and devices. You'll like the friendly staff, toll-free ordering, prompt service, and their selection of quality products. Here's their address:

BIOWELL CO.
P.O. Box 1448
Hermitage, PA. 16148
Call Toll-Free
1-800-877-2434
9 AM - 9 PM EST (M-F)

SUGGESTED READING

DIET, NUTRITION, AND CANCER
Committee on Diet, Nutrition, and Cancer
Assembly of Life Sciences, National Research Council
Published By:
National Academy Press
2101 Constitution Avenue NW
Washington, DC 20418

WHAT YOU CAN DO TO PREVENT CANCER
Oliver Alabaster, M.D.
Published By:
Simon & Schuster
1230 Avenue of the Americas
New York, NY 10020

CANCER, RISKS AND PREVENTION
Edited By:
M.P. Vessey, Professor of Social & Community Medicine
University of Oxford, and
Muir Gray, Community Physician
Fellow of Green College, University of Oxford
Published By:
Oxford University Press
Walton Street
Oxford, OX2 6DP
Great Britain

**"FATS AND OILS — The Complete Guide to Fats
and Oils in Health and Nutrition"**
Udo Erasmus
Published By:
Alive Books
Vancouver, B. C. V5W 3T1
Canada

INDEX

INDEX

cataracts - 46
cervical cancer - 8, 13, 17, 23,
    25, 37, 39, 59, 171-172
cesium - 196-197
Chauvin, Dr. Remy - 156-157
chemotherapy - 35, 40, 46-49,
    167, 174
    adriamycin - 47, 48
    circadian timing - 48-49
    cisplatin - 48, 49
    nausea - 47
    verapamil - 47
chemoprevention - 267-268
Chen, Dr. Jun-shui - 75
Chinese dietary study - 76
Chiodo, Dr. G.T. - 15
cholesterol - 54, 66-67, 76, 79,
    87, 89, 91, 156, 228
choline - 192-193
chondrosarcoma - 45
chordoma - 45
choroidal melanoma - 45
choriocarcinoma - 46
colorectal cancer - 11, 14, 23, 33,
    38, 39, 42, 55, 56, 58, 62,
    64, 65, 76, 127, 241, 266
Committee on Diet, Nutrition and
    Cancer - 53
Commoner, Dr. Barry - 71
Community Nutrition Institute -
    221-222
THE CONCEPT OF MIND - 178
Connor, Dr. William E. - 94, 97
copper - 248
cottage cheese - 110, 113, 115,
    118, 119, 122, 137, 143,
    145, 146-151, 191, 207, 246
cows' milk - 228-229, 246
cruciferous vegetables - 55-56
Cullen, Joseph W., Ph.D. -
    256-257, 259, 261, 267, 269
cytology - 39

D

Davidson, Dr. Michael - 93
Denny's Restaurant - 228
dental examinations - 15, 204,
    254
dequalinium - 29

DeVita, Dr. Vincent T. - 1
DHA (docosahexaenoic acid) -
    89-90, 92, 93, 95-99, 100
DHEA (dehydroepiandrosterone) -
    196
diet - 11, 12, 17, 52-78, 257
DIET, NUTRITION AND
    CANCER - 52
DIETARY GUIDELINES FOR
    AMERICANS - 236
DNA - 4, 5, 62, 193, 205
Duesberg, Peter H., Ph.D. - 3
Dyerberg, J., M.D., Ph.D. - 90-92

E

East West Foundation - 167, 170
EAST WEST JOURNAL - 170
Edelson, Dr. Richard - 29-30
EFA (essential fatty acids)
    102-104, 107, 108, 112,
    113, 115, 122, 126, 127,
    133, 140, 229, 250
ELF - 202
endometrial cancer - 11, 172-173,
    266
EPA (eicosapentaenoic acid)
    89-90, 92, 93, 95-99, 100,
    129
Erickson, Dr. Eric H. - 153
Eskimos - 91-92, 129
esophageal cancer - 8, 10, 11, 69,
    76, 230
estrogen - 65
extracorporeal photophoresis -
    29-30

F

Farber, E. - 192
fats - vii, 11, 17, 53, 54, 58, 64,
    65, 67-68, 79, 80, 81,
    93-94, 102, 103, 107, 108,
    109, 114, 116, 118, 120,
    125, 216, 226, 227, 235,
    236, 248, 266
FDA (Food and Drug
    Administration) - 80, 187,
    213-214, 217, 222, 224
fecapentaene - 57
Feverfew - 94

INDEX

INDEX

lumpectomy - 42
lung cancer - 8, 10, 15, 22, 23, 25, 30, 55, 59, 64, 76, 185, 200, 230, 265, 271
lymphatic system - 6, 12, 16, 121, 136
lymphoma - 30, 31

M

macrobiotic diet - 18, 162-174
macrophages - 26, 28, 53, 182
malignancy - 2, 5, 6, 20
mammography - 13, 17, 36, 37, 39
manganese - 245
margarine - 68, 81, 84-86, 104, 124
mastectomy - 42
Mayo Clinic - 61
melanoma - 28, 200
Mest, H.J. - 97
metastasis - 1, 2, 6, 7, 13, 16, 21, 34, 41
methionine - 192-193
Meyerhof, Otto - 108
Meyskens, Dr. F.L. - 239
micronutrients (see Vitamins and minerals) - 74-75
microwaves - 181-182
Miller, Dr. Jonas - 181-82
mitosis - 2
Moertel, Dr. Charles - 188
molds - 73
molybdenum - 245
monoclonal antibodies - 31-32
monostearates - 215
Morishige, Fukumi, M.D., Ph.D. - 60-61
Mormons - 64-65, 258
MSG (monosodium glutamate) - 215, 228
mucilage - 106
muesli - 142, 147-148
multiple myeloma - 8
mutagens - 4, 70-71, 72
mutation - 6

N

nabilone - 47

National Cancer Institute - vii, 1, 2, 3, 5, 8, 9, 11, 12, 13, 14, 16, 17, 26, 27, 28, 33, 36, 47, 48, 49, 53, 63, 156, 188, 196, 241, 252, 256-269
nausea - 47
Neuringer, M., Ph.D. - 97
Newbold, R.F. - 3
Nieper, Dr. Hans - ix, 188-190, 202
nitrosamines - 54, 69, 193, 215
NutraSweet® - 219, 220-222

O

oatmeal mash - 141
obesity - 63, 65, 107, 189, 236
oil 80-85, 104
    cold-pressed - 81
    hydrogenated - 84-85
    industry - 80-88
    refined - 82-84
    unrefined - 82
olive oil - 80, 105
omega-3 fatty acids - 92-96
oncogenes - 3, 4, 5, 200, 201
oncologist - 20, 34, 122
oral cancer - 10, 15, 16, 59, 230, 234, 265
oral contraceptives - 14
osteoma - 133
osteosclerotic sarcoma - 136-137
ovarian cancer - 11, 48, 173
Overell, R.W. - 3

P

PAH (poly-cyclic aromatic hydrocarbons) - 69, 70, 71
pancreatic cancer - 8, 10, 11
PAP test - 13, 17, 37, 39, 271
Pauling, Linus, Ph.D. - 61, 239
pesticides - 54
Peto, Richard - 58
Pflueger, Eduard - 107
phenylaline - 220
phosphorus - 249
photodynamic therapy - 30
Poland (fat studies) - 128-129
potassium - 246
potassium bromate - 216

INDEX

INDEX

U

ultrasound - 39
urea - 197
urinary tract - 12
URPs (unique radiolytic products)
    - 223-224
uterine cancer - 8

V

Vallera, Dr. Daniel - 32
Vanderpool, David M., B.S. - 56
verapamil - 47
visual imagery - 180
visualization therapy - 18, 176-184
vitamins
    A - 58, 59, 76, 105, 106, 161,
      191, 224, 238-239, 249,
      266, 267, 268
    B - 242-243
    C - 60, 61, 69, 76, 108, 224,
      239, 240, 245, 253, 266
    D - 62, 73, 105, 247
    E - 62-63, 83, 104, 105, 106,
      161, 224, 232, 242, 243,
      266
    P - (bioflavonoids) - 240

W

Wade, Carlson - 157
Warburg, Otto Heinrich - 108
weight (see obesity)
Weinberg, Robert A. - 3-4
Weiner, Michael A., Ph.D. - 99
Wells, I.C. - 192-193
Wilkins, Dr. Tracy - 57
Williams, Dr. R.J. - 254
Wurtman, Dr. Richard J. - 220

X

Xing, Dr. Mei - 193

Y

yin-yang concept - 162-165
Yoirich, Dr. Naum P. - 154
Yugoslavia (bee pollen studies) -
    155

Z

zinc - 54, 249-250

Index of Charts and Illustrations

Other Outstanding Books on Health And Natural Healing From Fischer Publishing

Miraculous Breakthroughs for Prostate Problems by William L. Fischer

Good news for every man who has prostate or occasional impotency problems. This new book describes in detail many of the latest therapeutic discoveries from Europe and America that can prevent, relieve or cure prostate disease, without the agony of prostate surgery. The book also discusses other male problems like testicle diseases, cancer, and the subject of impotency with honesty and sensitivity.

(Special Library Hard Cover Edition)
ISBN 0-915421-12-7 .... $18.95

The Miracle Healing Power Through Nature's Pharmacy by William L. Fischer

Now you can learn how to treat virtually every disease or condition known to man—naturally! A comprehensive guide to help you and heal you...the most complete...most useful...and most up-to-date work of its kind. Complete with many documented case histories and 32 full-color illustrations.

ISBN 0-915421-04-6 .... $19.95

Mysterious Cause Of Illness and How To Overcome Every Disease From Constipation to Cancer by Dr. Jonn Matsen, N.D.

Famed Canadian doctor uncovers the mysterious *REAL* cause of illness—and shows you how to overcome every disease from constipation to cancer. Dr. Matsen's acclaimed food-based "miracle cures" use *no* drugs, *no* surgery. They simply turn on the natural "internal healing poweer" built into every human body. Here is a safe, easy approach to health and longevity that has cured many "hopeless" cases after conventional medicine has failed! If you read nothing else, read Dr. Matsen's new revelations of secret remedies.

ISBN 0-915421-09-7 .... $16.95

The Romance of Creative Healthy Cookery by William and Trudy Fischer

We know you'll fall in love with this book, because over 800,000 European families already have. All of the recipes are either time-tested Eurpoean classics or inventive new dishes created by health minded experts and chefs. They have been adapted for ingredients that can be easily purchased at your local grocery store. Extra features include calcium-rich recipes to fight osteoporosis, nutritious vegetable dishes, budget meals fit for royalty and think lite...cook lite...eat lite receipes.

ISBN 0-915421-11-9 .... $18.95

How To Survive In The Hospital by Joan Haas-Unger, R.N.

There are too many procedures, performed by too many doctors, in too many places, with too high a stroke-and-death rate. This landmark book can help you lower your risks and increase your chances of survival in the hospital.

ISBN 0-915421-06-2 .... $12.95

Shipping/Handling $3.00 for one book.
Additional books $1.00 each.

Fischer Publishing
Box 368
Canfield, Ohio 44406
(216) 533-1232